GW01071734

NOTHING SACRED

VOLUME ONE

By Fatma Durmush

'One million people commit suicide every year'.
The World Health Organization

Published by:
Chipmunkapublishing
PO Box 6872
Brentwood
Essex
CM13 1ZT
United Kingdom

http://www.chipmunkapublishing.com

Edited by Gerry Deb

Front illustration © de Bùrca

Nothing Sacred is a two volume
anthology.
The second volume contains work by
Pam Wypych,
John Sheehy, and GS de Bùrca.

Nothing Sacred

This book started in a classroom, a friend suggested I write a diary, which I proceeded to do. The class enjoyed the two pages which I wrote, and I was encouraged to write more. But it was not all plain sailing, I suffer from schizophrenia and the voices would start every time I mentioned them.

I managed the voices, and there were oceans of pages. All the pages in the world to be written and I had to write those pages. Sometimes the book would deal with my family, and sometimes celebrity figures which the voices were fancying.

Both my parents are disabled, my father has cancer and we are managing on a shoestring. My father too is a schizophrenic, but his is a controlled schizophrenia, whereas mine is out of control. Doctors give me hope, but ever since starting university the voices have been very acute, and then we come to mental health. What is mental health?

If a doctor were to read this book he would think it a case study. It is a classic study of a paranoiac schizophrenia. It deals with the illness on a daily basis, and the wider aspect is the world of healthy people contrasted with the illness, and how the shadowy world is almost taking over from the real world.

Miss Beyaz is a real singer in Turkey whom I think readers would like, then there are other characters which are part of the neurosis. I changed their names, but some I have left as too fantastic to be taken seriously.

This book is a text on schizophrenia, it deals with mental health. This book is like a story of a mind, and the curing of the ailments and grievances of schizophrenia. Eventually I had to end the book because the pain of writing it became too much to bear.

I have been truthful and honest. Mentally now, I tread an acrobatic balance, sometimes the balance of my mind is not perfect, but then no one is perfect.

Fatma Durmush, 2005

13-02-03

Today there was a funny programme on Turkish television about men having two wives each, and the women being thankful that he doesn't divorce them. That is what the husbands say. There was some woman with a heart complaint and she did not want a divorce, her husband had another woman on the go and had gotten two children by her. The former wife had to be content with visits of two months apart. She now has a job and doesn't receive a penny, but what if I could work? I would give up the voice and his stinking ways, and be alone for the rest of my days. I am fed up to the teeth with the voice and his unfaithfulness. Don't ask me how a voice can be unfaithful, but he is, and he goes to massive detail as to his unfaithfulness. I must take my medication, because otherwise I'll go mad again.

I keep on wondering what to do, there is too much to read, I didn't read the newspaper today, and still I did not stop reading. I've read Louise MacNiece, he is a very difficult poet to get along with, the reason I find him difficult is, he uses imagery which is not immediately recognised, and one has to go over what he has written, my favourite poem is The Reflection. I found it in an anthology. I did not think much about his collection. I like Auden better, he is modern, but MacNiece has style and vim, which, if he had jazzed himself up and became less sober, and more autobiographical, would have helped him. I had no idea that Auden had been gay until I read his poems, but MacNiece, I don't know anything about him, and it is confusing me that I can read a whole book, and not be revealed anything, is that what, as poets we should do?

I'll be reading on the March 13th. I hope it will goes well and I have less to worry about, but then, what do I do all day but go to classes and try to write, sometimes my health gives out, and sometimes a terrible dislocation grips me. I have nearly written the essay and I am going to hand it in on Tuesday.

Tomorrow is Valentine's Day and I probably won't get a card. I have grown used to not being loved, and being a stinking idiot when it comes to men. The voice is there and while I type it types too, it won't put ideas into my head but suicide is not far off. I am tired of it all and wonder what to do.

My hair is white and I feel a burden on my soul, a terrible loneliness grips me, and I want to be someone more jolly, calm, and serene. I guess if it was not for my illness I could have done much with my life, but I did sell a painting. The school fees are nearly due and I had a row with mother the other day about it. She says I spend money like water, yet she was on the phone for one hour, and has sent a hundred pounds to my aunt who has just been widowed. It was my idea but I am not the only one who spends money.

My cousin works and apparently they don't pay him. What a jerk, he has joined the club of fools and beggars. I am not even worried he'll survive, it is auntie who won't. I hope she gets the money. I now do some voluntary work teaching the homeless how to write.

16-02-03

Already it is after February, and the months are speeding along in a busy enclave of work and food. Ziynet and Belgin came, Ziynet with her family. Little Ted wanted to stay and sleep in our bed, but they have now gone to their own house, and our house now is so quiet, I want to cry. Dad's bleeding has set me thinking about the nature of life and death. I wonder what death is like, it is an end, and a start of being dead, but that is all that is healthy to know.

Sadiye phoned, a cousin who lived with us, until I had had enough of her. She used to come every year and stay several months, then I had the bright idea of refusing her, and she went elsewhere and slept on floors. Now her sister is marrying a chemist researcher and they are coming to gloat. What petty things females are with their small minds!

Today passed in inactivity and plenty of washing up. I have come upstairs and typed my essay, and now I can breathe a sigh of relief. I best put my odds and ends in my bag and see what else I can do for tomorrow, it might snow, and if it does, mum can't go out. Her leg and her blood won't stand for it. She has artery thrombosis and has to take care. Belgin stayed today until about 5.30 P.M. She is such a lovable girl, she does listen, and looked all my sketch books. I have six.

I love my family and don't want to see them suffer; I hope they feel the same way too. I have to go.

22-02-03

So here we go again on this turnabout. Dad's cancer has recurred and the doctors said if he smokes, he'll die. His cancer is caused by his smoking and I don't want to say 'I told you so'. Ziynet wants to take him to a faith healer but dad doesn't believe in it. Neither do I. He is sixty eight and it has been a good life. I just can't bear the loneliness of mother when he goes. I imagine me and mum sitting and eating and talking until mum goes. Such is life.

Sadiye came yesterday with my books. The books which I had bought, and not read, were not in there.

Fatosh is getting married, she is marrying well. I think Sadiye was sad, and she has grown up. Then I went to Flora. She wants a quarter of a million pounds to fund her centre, and this person asked about the Copleston Centre, I said of course we want it to remain as a community hall, where worshippers come, where users come, where the entire world comes.

Then I had to rush to my college to do some amateur paintings. Some of the others could really paint, and I felt like I had a mop instead of the pastel. I am going to practice, though. One woman painted the nude as if she were Lucien Freud, and I want to do that, it is impossible that I am forty and so untalented. I placed all my art work to be judged, and I am not well pleased with my portfolio. I think I need to do more work. There is more to be done, always.

I sold two paintings but what does that mean? I am going shopping to buy some clothes and an apron, and a purse. I tore a fiver yesterday. It got stuck and I tried to pull it out and it came in two. I must relax, half term, and I can practice. I need to buy a sketch book.

26-02-03

I have bought the sketch book, and have been at the Tate to see Constable and Turner, and other 18th century painters. The Rape of the Deutschland, a simply massive painting, as big as the wall, impressed me; the simplicity of the design.
Everything was great, the way in which not many colours were used, to portray the soberness of the painting, was extremely creative. I then said

good bye to Gillian, and went to the cinema, and saw the Hours. It was as sober as a painting, but of course it was modern and more complex than the ship and survivors. I just enjoyed it. I came home and read Charlotte Salome's book. How she was killed by the Nazis when pregnant, and how she managed to finish her book, and it was just left for someone to find. I feel sorry for her, and thank Valerie for lending me the book.

I've still got to read the introduction and things, but I want to paint like her. Yesterday I did not read the paper. I missed it. On Monday I am leaving the computing class, it's not me. I can't think like that. Mum tried her best to persuade me to stay, but I just dread the basics of mathematics, and goggledook English.

Freedom to do what I want to do is going to my head. Today, I said I did not want Empire to send the washing machine, mum has been washing by hand for two weeks. I went and bought a machine at half price, which dad had said he knew of.

6-03-03

I'm trying to read Terry Pritchett. In the art group today I found myself trying to read Mills and Boon. I read a page and could not go any further. But I copied the picture, and Jaime said it was all right. I tried to kiss Sylvia on the cheek, and she gave me a full mouth sloppy, chaste kiss. I told mum, Sylvia is eighty eight. The voice did not object. Why is the voice trying and succeeding in making me have sex with women? But I must be calm because I can out wit the voice, it is me after all. I don't believe that a man can behave in such a disgustingly high handed, and stupid, manner. I have wasted my life. I know no peace, if I'm not arguing with the voice in my head, I am in deep trouble with someone else. I don't like it. This lurking about, this patience, what is it? Why? If I should die in the attempt to be a woman, then so be it. At least I attempted it.

There is John, who I think fancies me, but I don't think it possible, knowing my circumstances, and I think he drinks. He is also younger than me and I don't want a toy boy. The voice won't let me near him. But as I rage, I feel my blood pressure rising. A terrible quietness has invaded me, making me go overboard. I am asexual and I prefer it.

The quietness of night, many die in the night time, and not see anything but black night. I, a virgin, have all the world to look at, and I go throwing it on a voice, because of the voice's glib tongue.

I am handicapped because of my abuse, I can't use the computer and rely on the voice, I can't cook and I can't be anything but creative. The voice is non creative, yet he is beginning to edit my things. Now where do I come in? My split personality is such that I can't breathe. I need the voice to do all the practical things, so that I can do all the creative. But to be creative I need the practical. Do I sound mad? I must be. Father isn't smoking, and he is always demanding attention like a baby from mum. Mum is patience itself, when she loses patience I go into the kitchen, I can make a cup of coffee, no problem.

Our neighbour's child has leukaemia. She's only two. My nephew David has one weak eye, but we are thankful it wasn't worse. David has stayed with his mum this week because the teachers are on strike in his school, and Ziynet says he has been a good boy. He is not eating, though. Belgin has invited me to go on a holiday with her and Roger. She's paying, all I have to pay for is the flight, and I think I can manage that. I just have to shift around dates. I don't know if I can make it in May. We are going to Italy. I don't mind Italy, if it is Roger's family, there will be lots of food and lots of pitying glances. I want to see Rome and the El Grecos, and the huge collections. I know that Roger and Belgin will chose a mountain and climb it, and they will wash their feet in the stream and generally be active. I am moaning, but I hate climbing mountains.

10-03-03

Today I have been enormously busy doing nothing. I went to the doctor with dad and told them that he is bleeding. Then went shopping, and later took Susie to the vet. I think the vet is not busy, so I have done other things. I was on the phone to the gallery about mounting an exhibition, but don't know if it is going to be a solo or joint one. I think it'll be joint, I haven't got a lot of paintings worth exhibiting, and Sylvia is 89, so this might be her last chance. I am thinking of getting Roger as well in on the act. On Monday I am going to see the place, and will know if it is worth it. They do all the publicity and it is only 200 pounds, and they have space in August. So I am ready if they are. The Big Issue will send me cheques for my writing. I have finished one sketch book. I phoned the Fellowship and asked for space to put my pictures in, I need to go there and scan things in. I'm going to phone them on Friday. Then I went overboard and phoned about the university, and also on the phone about mother to the doctor. So I got in a stew because everything came all at once. I bought dad some steaks, liver and kidneys. He said he felt dizzy and I am worried. If he dies we'll be alone, and he has his uses. Mum and I will miss him if he dies. I did some typing, had a bath and skimmed the paper. Now I am tired. I feel very half formed, as if my head was not my own. Dad did something silly, he stopped his insulin and when the nurse checked it was 23. The machine was not working properly.

13-3-03

Today I read Nothing Sacred, my diary, or rather Gerard read it for me. It was well received. Everyone laughed, and to be successful in a form I enjoy writing, is great. Yesterday I edited Fabini's play, I think her plays are excellent, quite unlike her other stuff, which is poor. The book yesterday was hard and demanding, I lost some material, all

Dan's work. I think it has been tampered with, but what does one do? Go to the police and I am being paranoid. I am still reading Pritchett, Mike said it was his first three books which are great. I hope I am reading the right books, I am enjoying the novel. Hope to go on holiday soon, then I can be rested and refreshed, ready to face whatever.

Brief good news, dad might live for some time, we don't know exactly how long. He might live longer than what we thought of as months. I am seeing the doctor on Monday with Ziynet and Belgin. Ziynet made mum cry because she was upset, and they both said things which simmered over. Well, anyway Ziynet said it was Mum's fault that she did not go to hospital to see the doctors, forgetting that mum has only one leg, and she ran on and on.

They seemed to have calmed down today. Mum and I had a conversation which illustrates she can be so stupid when it comes to politics. I said something to the effect that Denktash is after what he can keep, because he has a car, and a lovely place to live, so doesn't care if the rest of the population are starving. Mum, being pro Denktash, hotly denied this, saying that he was a great leader. So if he is a great leader, why is he so stubborn? He keeps on saying the same words, and he won't listen to reason. Mum began to scream, so I left her to it.

My feet smell. I have smelt my feet all day and it is giving me an inferiority complex. I saw Brian today. He looked well fed, and he has lost that haunted expression which I liked, he said he had money and I think he fancied a bit of fun and games. I wonder if he loved me once. He certainly helped me, suggesting I paint and draw. We caught up on our news then I had cold feet. I haven't felt so vulnerable for a while. We seemed to be talking about how much my hair has changed, and I wanted to say let's talk about something else. But you know when Brian wants to be rude he can be. We had not spoken because the voice in my head had stopped it. Now it is because Brian has hardened towards me, I think it is a reflex reaction. I got scared because my feet smelt, and the time was dragging, making a mountain of my eating an egg sandwich and rhubarb. I sometimes wonder if I am a woman or a child. What will I do when Mum dies? I also read the poem Besime Walks, it was well received, though Maurice has seen faults in it, and Michael said, for he had not seen the first draft, that it was confusing. This Michael is a talented poet, not the first Michael. He really can write poems and I respect his criticism, so I changed it to clarify it, in case other people are confused. I haven't written much, but what I write I want to be good quality writing.

15-03-03

I keep on remembering what Brian had said, and going over him in my own mind. I definitely think he hates me. He is much colder, more glossy, right down to his paintings. He now does graphic art and I remember him doing oil portraits. Did I call him to come to me? Anything is better than the voice, the days speed past, and I am both waving and drowning. The days are jewels, ready to be made into something. Today I did the questions which I will ask Roger. Yesterday, Big Issue's Theo phoned, he said he was interested in publishing my 'mother' article. Yesterday I did not go out, I had my injection, and talked to this old woman of ninety two who thought I was in my twenties, early thirties, and I was so frank it shocked her. I told her my age and things about the household, my father being terminally ill. My own illness I hinted at, but in the end she did not offer me a job. Her daughter in law wanted a typist and she had offered me an interview. I now realize I would not have got it. My despair is complete.

The voice in my head says he has a new telepathic girl friend; I am so disgusted and amused that I don't know what to say. The voice is crowing and it is wearisome. I am weary, I am tired. I took the dog for a walk and that calmed me. Suzy was jumping and bouncing about. You know once I actually believed the voice had been a man. Now I am in the world of the real and it is killing me. I am a prime fool. Even if the voice is real his character is despicable. He acts in a purely selfish way. He loves no one but himself, and I am fed up with being a vehicle for him.

My nurse has gone on holiday and left me to cope on my own, but he did not even phone me, and I am on my own coping with my illness and my parents. Mum is saving money so she won't spend on anything but essentials. Father did not give us any money, but mum always gets careful when alone, and she has already buried dad in her mind, so she is saving money.

19-03-03

Dad isn't going to die. Thank the Lord, now we can continue with our lives where we left off. War has started, terrible thing. A cold shudder went through me, there is this war and I don't want it. Good news about dad came on the 17th. My sisters went to Mr Cetti and asked him. He definitely has cancer but they don't know how far it has spread. It, apparently, is not even prostrate cancer, bladder cancer, it is just on the surface.

My days pass in a haze of anger and suspicion. I am almost suicidal, and I want to end my life when I know I'll go with dignity. The voice is making my life into hell. I want to get away from the voice but can't. He can't see women, every woman he sees, he wants me to chat them up, to be a man to them, just because he is having a ball, or thinks he is. Each day I die and become a bag lady, which the voice says I am. As the days become more and more attuned to the voice, I keep on going over the same old ground, and I think it is best that I leave the voice alone. Think of something else. But every time I sit next to a woman the voice rears his ugly neck, I want to be left alone to see what I'll do, but it is always the voice's demands, I am through with it. I want to end it, but when and how? God give me courage to go on, I know it is wrong to commit suicide but I feel so bitter and used up.

So daily my misery grows, I can't walk happily, I feel the voice looking for women. It is like having a dog which is on heat, and it is embarrassing with the dog all over the place. There was this woman who had a dog, which was older than 10, and he had gone like that. The voice reckons he has a 22 year old as a new girl friend, and wants me all hitched up with a woman. But I AM NOT GOING TO BE. I prefer to die.

20-03-03

Today I went to class, painting, and creative writing. Murray Rowland was there. Murray is the head of humanities at Morley College. He is having a book out after, he says, submitting it thirty times. The war is on, and the group talked about a man with a gas mask reading a paper. The papers had something about the water supply and how important it is to have canned food. Mum is going tomorrow to buy these things, I think I'll go with her and buy things for myself as well, I need some paper and art materials. I got paid a lot of money this week. I received 130 pounds from Mary Ward, 30 from the Big Issue and 20 from Jaime. I put the 130 pounds away and spent the rest on supplies, art supplies.

Today he voice said he depended on me. I don't think he means to be cruel but he is, one moment he can talk me into a good mood and the next moment I am miserable. Not that I am not miserable often, but the voice aggravates my misery and makes me vulnerable. I waited for Brian Williams, the man who said he loved me, and sure enough he did not come. He must think I am old. He has got definitely more opinionated, and determined on hurting me which he never did before. He used to think the world of me, and now it is as if I have ceased to be what he wants. He wants someone young, like all men. I feel so bloody old.

Two people read today and they both had entertaining stories to tell. I especially liked the one about the sixties and how the hippies went on a peace march. It was about two pregnant women and their spouses. Joan seems to know what she is writing about. She has a deft hand. I compared the piece to Mrs Dalloway. Mike Walker compared it to Tolstoy's Death of Ivanich which he is adapting as a radio play.

I found a play group which I am going to approach tomorrow. I hope I have luck with them. So another day has been done, and another jewel. These days are so precious, like jewels in my crown.

23-03-03

I remember things which happened nearly thirty years ago as if they had happened yesterday. I remember how I got my glasses. Erturk hit me on the head so severely that I thought I had gone blind. I sat on my bed blinking. He was laughing at me. He hit me again a couple of times because a man had pinched my bottom in the lift. Erturk did not like it. He hit me repeatedly when mother and father were in the hospital, and he had sole charge of us. Or rather, I was in charge. By the time he finished I needed glasses desperately. I felt vulnerable, so I sat in bed and thought what I needed was protection from him, if he felt that way about me attracting men, then the best way not to attract men was to wear glasses, besides my eyes were weak. They had been weak before, but with the onslaught they grew weaker.

Back to today, the voices have calmed down, and the lesbian proposition seemed to have settled. I have begged the voice that we can be like brother and sister, even if he likes me not. He wants to go off somewhere with someone else, probably get married, but how, when he inhabits my body and my space, I don't know. Any way, the voice is getting restless. All day it used to say 'what will happen to you when I am gone', and I was figuring out that of course he can't go, because he is, after all, a voice. Anyway today we had a peaceful day listening to the radio and working in the garden, and generally doing things calmly and collectively. Tomorrow is another day, and I think the voice is meeting someone else on Tuesday, as a sweetener he said he can't be bothered with me. So in a way we are a married couple, with the husband after a younger version of himself.

I know I am getting old. I have my period and it is not as bloody as it used to be. I am drying up.

I told my nurse all this but he tends to ignore the voice, which I like, some people just love the voice, they can listen to me going on about him. Mother is well in pain. Her leg is hurting, and dad smells of blood and urine, they are not happy, and I am remembering how I got my glasses and we are not happy. This household is not happy. Even the voice is not happy, we are a miserable lot. Dad will have his operation in a fortnight. Sunday the 6th. I know he is nervous but he has to have it. I best go downstairs for a rest. I have been typing G. Campbell's stuff, and I like her work, shows promise. I am also reading Conrad, it is so stark and alive, I want to write like that, if I ever become an artist I think I want to become stark and alive. I want to write a great work and see it in print, and get recognition, not just money but recognition. I know I print things and have them published, but I want to be published by some big publishing house like Faber and Faber. I dream on.

24-03-03

Tonight I watch as others make their dreams come true. The lover of the voice was there, glorious and alive, I thought she was suffering in rage about something and wished not to know. It is better not to know of these things, and the voice did not want me to see the programme, he said he was through with the femme fatale. But I am dead, my summer is burnt out and my old age is creeping. Then mum and dad had a severe argument about the war. Dad said mum did not know about anything, and why was she watching the news. Mum replied, "I want to learn." The dog watched with interest and I tried to calm them down. Dad thinks he will be in hospital on the 28th, so I explained yet again that he will not be, that it is only a check up.

Then I was in a rage, mum did not buy me towels, I called her a greedy so and so. She thought I called her a greedy whore. I shouted, and told her not true that I had called her any such thing, that went on for quite a while with mum in tears and dad sitting silent. Then I thought it was like Throw Momma off the Train, so I have come to write it all down, but feel so shattered that I could not read Conrad. The writing was jumping up and down, there were the good sentences, the writing so pure and great, but the reader was a jerk.

The voice has calmed down and now I am ready for bed, the day has been interspersed with highs and lows. We went shopping, and then I heard the afternoon play in the garden, about teachers kidnapping the education secretary's son and not holding him to any ransom, but to teach him a lesson. Then the tables are turned, and Barry (the boy) teaches the teachers a lesson, even mending the car and saving the suicidal teacher's life.

I want to write a play but there is no incentive to do so, I am so tired of waiting for the radio people I have given up hope. Any way I must write something.

26-03-03

Yesterday was a nightmare. I got up, had breakfast of weetabix and rushed to get to my class. I went as far as Kings Cross. Saw the barriers and went to the next platform which an impatient Guard pointed me to. Everyone one of us packed good and proper like sardines. Then some stupid person left their bag, so off the train we came again. I went to the wrong bus stop, waited for ten minutes, and then asked someone, "Across the street!" Again we were jam packed on the bus, and the sirens calling were a distant murmur. Then I got lost in Holborn, and finally I was in my class. An hour late and feeling tipsy. I finished a sculpture class and then enrolled for print making and more sculpture. At the graphic art class Rosemary was eating a cake, and Gillian was eating a cake, I was trying not to look at them. Valerie the teacher liked my monoprints; I was calm and happy for a change.

After class Rosemary and Gillian came with me to the station. Rosemary started to blow her whistle and the Station Manager came and spoke to her. He warned her not to whistle. Gillian and I did not speak. She said the Queen was a stupid cow and was not the right sovereign, anyway, it lasted for five minutes and I did not speak, nor Gillian. Then she was peeved because we had not spoken and said, "Thank you ladies for helping me!" Well I was not going to be put in jail. That got me thinking how many people do something for others, Rosemary is my hero, but I think she does it because she is frustrated she can't work. She sustained a back injury. Gillian and I went to the Jubilee line all the way from Russell Square, and the voice is saying things like this is your mate, this is it.

I got rid of Gillian, and started to be jam packed like sardines again. The Jubilee Line had something wrong with it and there were delays, you know, "normal travelling arrangements". Then I went home and had a bite to eat, earlier, at college, the lasagne was too salty, I was so thirsty. Anyway today I am going to teach.

27-03-03

So I taught, rather I wrote a ten minute play. I was taken advantage of, but I think I am always being taken advantage of. Fabini has got 10,000 pounds to do a video, I supplied the script and she hasn't even offered me money. Joseph came, he was found in a very compromising position with his father's dead body and I can feel his guilt. Every time he opens his mouth he is guilty, but it might be my imagination. Then John came, I don't know his life story, I asked him what he would do to a woman he had grown tired of? Would he tell her straight or would he lie to her, procrastinate? He said he was too soft and could not. Well I think that is bullshit, and that is how arguments, murders happen.

The voice yesterday was awful. He compares me to gay characters and thinks he knows me. I can't help being older. Today I wanted to die so much that it hurt. Every step that I take is a burden. But today the voice was quiet, and when I said I didn't want a smelly old woman fucking me, it gave me images of young women. Then I said I did not want a sister fucking me. It was nonplussed. Then my heart began playing up. It hurt so much. The voice feels quite separate from me and I am always in the wrong with it. I did not realize that it did not like me until this year. The voice just goes on and on. Yesterday I heard a play on the radio and then I saw Rehab, a violent documentary-like drama. I realize that I have been lucky in avoiding drugs, but food is a drug too, and that's what is killing me. I had chocolates and quite a few biscuits about ten. The voice is quiet, waiting for my next move, like I am waiting for his, and it is a waste of my life to be fucked and cuddled by something I can't even see.

The voice doesn't want a man fucking me because he says he is not gay, and I don't want a woman fucking me because I say I am not gay, so there is this impossible position in which I find myself. I feel suicidal and I want to talk to my nurse.

I wrote a funny piece tonight called Mabel, and I am having it read next week. My review was read out in class and everybody clapped, it was a moment which made me feel proud. I am proud to be a writer, proud to have had all this, and proud because I have talent. No matter how I live I'll always be proud of myself, because that is who I am, proud to be a victim. I am proud of myself because no one can tell me any different, not even the voice.

Rosemary did not speak to me today and I am glad because she is too rash, and after the whistle blowing incident she thinks I am a fraud. I know I am a fraud; I don't need to be told. I am the world's greatest coward. I am not going to be put in jail for a crime. No way, why the voice would crow in amazement and be ever so superior, besides I don't fancy being in jail with all those people who've done terrible things, and been traumatized by themselves and their families. I want a normal life with a normal man and not the voice. Mike says I am the most miserable person on the planet. But consider this, what do I have? I have nothing but my talent and a bit of cash. I have a given place, I must do something to free my mind from this oppression, only I can't, and my victim is me.

I saw Jaime today and we discussed the grant application, he wanted me to give him the catalogue which I did, then Jennifer said take it back, if he loses it you've had it. I took it and told Jaime I would photocopy it for him. I think I'll phone Jackson and get him a copy. He said he would hire the hall to me for 150 pounds a week. That is good news, because if the exhibition costs more than two thousand I would not have been able to do anything but count chickens.

I will have twenty six paintings and they will be exhibited in June or August, apparently a dead period. Sylvia, my co exhibitor will also have twenty five paintings, and I think I'll exhibit some of my sketch books and sculpture. Father has his appointment tomorrow, and I fear tomorrow, I fear that I'll forget I have a tutorial at five and just go and sleep forever. The cats are fighting and it is time I went to bed.

Kerry read a brilliant short story today and my admiration and respect knows no bound. Mike Walker and she have a rapport which only a gifted writer and her teacher can have. She said *promptly* and Mike Walker heard *portly.* It went on for weeks and weeks, then Kerry was attacked. She was nearly strangled and fainted. Her jewellery was stolen. Life can be terrible, even for rich people. Her husband was not there. I think she is getting over it now, but I find her work is not up to her usual standard. It is deeper, fuller, yet it lacks that playfulness, that essence which she can have. I really must leave writing, I feel like I can bask in the company of my word processor for a bit more. Words just flow and everything is right with the world.

28-03-03

I have had a busy day. Dad had an appointment, so I took him in a cab to Queen Elizabeth hospital, urine test, blood test, cardiac test, blood pressure test. We did not even have time to drink our coffees. We eventually found the interpreter. Mrs Ayshe gave us some leaflets, and then left us as we made our way to the canteen to sample the delights of sandwiches. "Two tuna sticks with a cup of coffee and a coke." A black woman bought three chicken sticks and the man said "Please will help." No it won't, nothing helps the over worked canteen waiter or waitress, trust me, I know. I finished my meal first and put the packets into bins, dad began gulping his coffee so I suggested we take it with us. We left the canteen and made our way to the car section. Old people, without a smile in their body, alone and uncared for, sat, in immobile silence. They could not hear, and they could not do anything but think. One was younger than the others, but they all blended in.

It was a terrible warning for giddy youth of what lies in store for them. "Durmush?" So we boarded the ambulance and went in style to our home. "Bloody women drivers." as two cars stood in our way. No one dared to contradict him. The ambulance driver's power was total, and he knew it. But he drove quickly and we made our way home.

"Good bye, thank you!" I said. But I did not want to offend, so said nothing when he looked cross and bored.

Went home and had a cup of tea with relish, then Pat came, the woman who walks our dog. "Stella bit another dog and your Susie ran off and waited for her at the gate. Stella needs to be muzzled; I isn't walking Stella unless she is muzzled. It's a dog pack and they won't let anybody else into their pack. Susie snaps but she doesn't bite, it is all too heart breaking."

"Mother's day on Sunday, you should do the cooking?" Why does everybody think I don't do anything? I go to classes, and I do my own thing, that is why. Afterwards Pat calmed down. Pat walks the dog, she has been doing so for the past 18 months or so, and we would be sorry if she did not walk the dog. I hope Susie behaves herself or we muzzle her.

I rang the advice line on cancer, about getting a grant and was offered nothing concrete. Bereavement and things were discussed. Went to college, I had an appointment with Rebecca about my essay. Spoke non-stop as my essay was corrected, but first had to ring Martin about some leaflets and posters and invitations to the exhibition, which might happen if we get the grant. Afterwards we went to art class and did some pictures. I also did a machete which I'll tear down next week. It took twenty minutes to make and it was someone living in a shoe.

Came home and heard about the hijack and the bombing of Kuwait. The war might be postponed or something. Maybe mum misheard. If it is then Bush is totally stupid and a coward. He starts and doesn't finish, he must be the most unpopular president ever. In the school canteen there is a picture of him, and we discussed that BUSH is doing everything he can for world peace and such. Satire is a good tool in war. Then I sat next to a black woman on the train and she took exception to my bag. Her satire ran as follows. "I was admiring your bag, rheumatology on it, are you a rheumatologist?" "No, I write for the Big Issue and they gave me the bag." I got out of her way, she spoke about onions in Holborn station, and how starving she was. I did not speak, for I had no desire to open my wounds, where I came from, what I did. No desire at all.

But the voice was saying she spoke to you, go for it, a romance. Fucked off real proper, I went on a bus and a woman sat close to me. I felt comfortable and slept. Then she got really close, so I edged nearer the window and she began to speak to herself, and, eventually sleeping and waking, she left the bus. I realized that I would never be cured, that this shit will go on and on forever. And forever is a long time.

31-03-03

The kids descended on us on Saturday while I was at college, when I got in they were in the bedroom, and they did not sleep until midnight. The clocks went forward, so it was midnight. We were heartily sick of one another. I took David to the park on Sunday and the poor chap enjoyed it. He was called clever and liked it. I am so glad I still remember how he asked for a cake. He was a severe and young looking boy. Leyla got on my nerves with her crying and the way she thinks she is a young girl instead of a child. That girl is so silly, yet one can't judge a six year old. Ted played football so I took him to the park. The brothers elected to go separately. We went to the sweet shop, but Leyla was crying, and wanting her mummy, so she did not go, I did not know what to do with her, or why she was crying, she said that Ted hit her and Ted swore he did not. Amazed at these children, especially since the other night they fell asleep at midnight. I was going to wash them at twelve. I gave them milk to drink, talked to them, then they fell asleep. I love them all, but I think they don't love me as much as they used to do, they did love my poem Situation is Bad by Hasan Huseyin which I translated, they liked the way everything is made better, I told a fairy story and they wanted more and more.

Someone contacted me about putting some of my poems into a book. I am pleased, then I got some money for a short article on mother. I'm thinking of spending it on Photoshop which comes to forty quid. I don't know when next I'll be paid or published, so today I spent a great deal on things which I need. I bought a small portfolio, then an A1 portfolio. I have to look smart for the interview. My cat has begun to scratch my portfolio and I don't think she'll stop.

Tomorrow I'm going to my sister's to look after the kids, we are going to school at 8, then Ziynet can go for her interview, and I can go on to the Big Issue. All this will take place on April 2nd. Tomorrow is April fool's day, and I never do a thing but cower on April fool. Apparently a long time ago April fool's day used to be New Year's Day. I read it in the Newsletter of the Big Issue. I thought my article had been better than it is. But what can one say, one writes, then offers it, and then falls out of love with it.

The Big Issue men think I am good looking, I can't believe that, after years of being told I am ugly, I felt like hugging everyone, today I went to get my money, and I saw them all in the street smoking, and we all chatted. I think money inhibits people. Then the good news, Gerry is going to do a poster for me. I must now do the poster because Gerry needs it by Wednesday, he is waiting for me to do it.

2-4-03

Gerry did not turn up. I babysat, Ziynet and I discussed her portfolio till one, and then I went to bed exhausted. Ziynet was hyper because she was harassed by interview nerves. I was wearing a thin summer coat and I was freezing, the day was cold and Leyla said, as she stood in the playground, that she was freezing too. I was baby sitting and loved every moment of it. I searched everywhere for a hanky to wipe David's nose, then found one and triumphantly began wiping his nose. He gave me a kiss. I am so proud of my sister's children. Then Ted said his friends were coming so could I leave him alone. I did not argue with the male pride, I don't want Ted to be suffering from school bullies. Then Leyla said could I leave her alone and she haughtily stared, at six she is a madam. I was left with David who was in line just like Ziynet said, then, I found he had disappeared behind a young woman whom Ziynet said would fetch him. I stood by for a while, mortified that I was alone without the kids. They had given me warmth and comfort and now they were gone.

I took a bus to Barking and this old man came and sat on my lap. Well almost. Then from Barking I went to Victoria and then to Vauxhall. I thought I would call about my father's holiday. He needs it after the operation. I phoned a lot, I spent two hours on the phone in the Big Issue, and then I thought I'd go and do some work on Photoshop. I needed my images enlarged for the course. I have an interview next week and I am as nervous as can be, it could mean doing the same old things, or if I get to university it could mean me being an artist.

Then Tom came and we had a party. We spoke about art and literature, and specifically the Maids, which I have never read. He said my play was similar, but he was puzzled about certain details which he would write to me about. We spoke about the radio plays; I don't think he was totally ignorant that we had signed an agreement to say nothing for one year. So I said nothing. Then Tom bolstered this guy and I bolstered him, and he came up with amazing jokes. I was so amused about a pregnant woman and her husband that I sent it off with my thing to BBC3 TV. The Big Issue did say they were running a competition but I had no time to refine it, and they would need it by the date of the interview, anyway I sent it off, typed and sealed. The Big Issue sent me a message which I deleted. I deleted the number which they gave me and I feel very much like a jerk. I think I have a phone phobia because I just can't stay on the phone tomorrow for an hour. Not like today. Then I got home from writing the jokes at six thirty and I was frozen and very thirsty. I am still thirsty. I must go downstairs and get something to drink.

3-04-03

I am still thirsty because I went to a class room party. Michael was there and he gave me my work. I was pleased. I read something, or Mike read everyone's stories, and we were all satisfied with ourselves. I had a busy time with the art group, we are applying for a grant to do the exhibition, and Jennifer said she'll type my application, but I am worried because we still haven't done the business plan.

I read the paper and then went upstairs to do work on the book. When I opened the disk it had squiggles and things, it was 241 pages. Men are so childish, why did he not say he refuses to edit it, instead of destroying my work? He is sixty, not a child. Any way I am glad I did my own editing with the college. Men! Does one need them? Anyway I'm not giving him anymore work to do.

I am ever so upset and mortified that he was doing that to my work, I feel violated. How dare he, luckily I have plenty of copies.

Spite is a crime against humanity, and I had actually begun to feel something, well no more do I feel like that. I hate sneaky people who destroy work. He destroyed months of work. I had edited and edited, refined and refined the work, so it was totally different to what he had, but still it would have been a good book with his help. Well I don't need anyone to help. How dare he do that to me, he must hate me a lot and I despise him for it. How dare he do that, and give me the disk as if he was offering me the world. The sneak, I feel violated. How dare he.

I wish this fly would go away, it has been pestering me since I sat on this damn computer, and I am feeling a little of the strain of being a woman and a writer, this fly is the last straw in my week. I got my work from the photos hot, I asked them how much a poster would cost and the man said 19 something pounds. Do they think I am made of money?

Do I use people? The voice has been complaining that he does all the work and I just reap the benefits, so he wants me to write a play about what he fancies. I don't know if I'll write the play, I don't fancy the girl the voice does. It is all getting a bit salty. I feel like laughing and crying, all at the same time.

Now it's stopped. The voice reckons the girl has had lesbian sex, so has gone off her. He says he'll pay money to her and be a jolly uncle figure. The voice has begun to criticize my dress and how I look. He says I look terrible. I reckon all women over the age of forty should not be wearing sleeveless, backless dresses. But that is what the voice wants me to wear, strapless dresses. My tits hanging loose, and me a wonder bra fan.

Anyhow that is what has been happening. I can't see women without thinking about the days and days which have been torture. Now I can think about my interview. We did mounting in college at the weekend. We did a lot of work and had a mock interview which went off well. I must have scared the daylights out of them, they said I did not show nerves. Mum and Pat had an almighty row, so Pat is not coming to walk the dog. She had hinted that she wanted more money. It seemed like too much effort for Pat, then I told her to walk the dog on Sunday, and mum bargained with another woman for two pounds, and the woman told Pat. I was nearly screaming today, saying I have to walk the dog forever or until I die. Then I washed the little girl, and she was so loveable that I just loved her, and don't mind the exercise. It will help me wear the strapless dress, if I ever do wear it. Ziynet's husband Ted is doing camping and it is freezing, I hope they are all right. I phoned Ziynet and Belgin about the holiday we are planning, and she said it was too soon, that all flights to Turkey and Cyprus have been cancelled. I don't think she is all that well, so I am a bit concerned.

I'm reading Freida's diary which I think is awfully interesting because she used text and images to portray pain. I have a pain in my joints, not unbearable pain, but I know it is cold outside and I feel it. After walking the dog, I went and saw some modern painters today in Tate Britain. I also went to the Big Issue to collect some art work, they are so near each other that I did both. I bought Frieda (Kahlo) for twenty quid, so expensive but invaluable. I must remember to take to college Charlotte Solem's diary. Mum found Freida very scary. I like the colours in it, and the essay about her life is interesting. She was not massively educated yet she had something, a weird power. I haven't seen the film, but if I do it will be worth it, I took out 60 pounds today and I am getting quite short. I bought a rucksack for 19 pounds, it is a good one. I bought the book and had a sausage roll and water, then I escaped the Tate. I went to Canary Wharf as well, and saw all the rich people buying things which we ordinary folk cannot afford. I did feel like buying a rucksack for 64 pounds, but the red thing I brought was better. I must get dressed, and go to bed. No, I am not naked, I am just dressed in my informal attire. I wonder how much longer the voice will stay.

12-04-03

I had the interview, I think I blew it, but my sister got in for the post graduate course. Did I blow it? I went there laden with my triplex and portfolio and several sketchbooks. It took me half an hour to get to the other side of the corridor, but finally I managed it. Went into the lift, went to the first floor. A woman helped me, turned out she was interviewing, I thanked her. Then she interviewed me, then a male came and interviewed me, but before that, they left me alone in the room for five minutes. I called Tracey Emin not a whore. I said she was way out. Then I went downstairs, the woman again helped me. I went downstairs into the phone box, called the taxi that had got me there. I stood trembling for a bit, did it go off well? I don't think it did. I don't think I got in. But hope eternal springs. They know about the voice, we spoke about it. I filled in the forms for the grant money. I am waiting.

Today the voice said a bizarre thing, I think the voice is deeply in love this time. The voice asked if he should screw me. He said I was too old to be a virgin. Well, bless me, that is a new thing. Terribly new. The voice has been selfish, obnoxious, and has made me sick for the past twenty years and now he is selfless. I know he no longer fancies me, there is nothing there to fancy, except for images in my head, and I am feeling so tired of it all. The other day my nurse saw me for two hours. I must be sick then. The nurse saw me and I saw the nurse, but it is me who has to live with this ailment. The voice is involved with this beautiful creature, he is totally besotted, but I think she is too young for him. I could self harm, I get up and it is there in the voice's gait. Get out, for I am involved with somebody else.

I am a burden in my own body. What kind of a life is that? When I am a burden to all and sundry?

But life goes on. I tried to listen to the Reith lectures, fell asleep and then woke to find them having a question or two, then fell back to sleep. All I know is that they were talking about the mind; even graduates were amazed at the man's inspiring awe. I have read INCEST by Marquise De Sade. I felt like reading an adult book, I was not even shocked. It is television that makes us unshockable. Tomorrow I am starting to read another book by Conrad, Heart of Darkness. I had read Graham Greene, but not with any attention. I could not get the references to the Catholic criticisms. All I knew is, it was about two people, and the husband was having an affair and could not get a divorce. Maybe that was all that there was to it, but in Marquise De Sade's tale I found the naughty bits convincing, his repentance and redemption utterly unconvincing. I think he did not repent. That Marquise De Sade who wrote the little book in prison was not a repentant sinner. He glories in wickedness. If only I had a wicked bone in my body.

The voice and me are through, really there is no such man as a man who is involved with one as young as his daughter. I used to read that these things happen to people, they fall out, but we had fallen out 21 years ago. Apparently the voice fell out of love with me when I French kissed Angel, and I am glad because Angel was the one for me. He was the only man who did not drag everything out. Then there was this chap who went to France and never came back. Apparently, he did not love me either, and who loves me any way? Who cares? Nobody loves me except my cats and dog and family. Sometimes they appear to be enough. But when I go to bed and cry myself to sleep I am alone, and that is the aloneness of destitution, despair grips my heart, and a terrible fear that I might end my days totally alone. The voice knew the baloney, and the voice knows how to drag the years and make grey hairs.

We went to the Chinese restaurant today and had a Chinese meal. We enjoyed talking to each other, Belgin, me, dad and mum, and Roger Belgin's partner. Belgin paid and I rushed and did some shopping. Susie stole a ball today and I rushed after her, and she was nearly run over by a car. She just would not give me the ball. Then she grew tired, so she did. The woman whose dog it was that had the ball came after us, and then gave up and disappeared. I went and bought Susie two balls. But I felt totally out of temper with Susie, she could have died. The woman did not collect the ball. Then when we were going to the Chinese I saw the neighbour who knew her, and told her about the ball, but she was talking to someone and snubbed me. But you should have seen me shouting at my dog, right in the middle of the street.

When I calmed down and read the newspaper mum said I was jealous of Belgin, and I am not, I am grateful to Belgin, and would like everyone to know that she is sane and well and I am not. That she has a life and I ruined mine. Why should I be jealous when she does all that she could to make my life better. I feel like a jerk. I am a jerk, but I can't help that.

13-04-03

Today has been a funny old day, with washing the endless piles of dishes and being active in housework, gardening and such. We planted some plants, forget me nots. I cried while I did the dishes and wished I might die. Today the voice was very rude and of course it wants Miss Beyaz. A Turkish star whom it says gave up her virginity to him. I am mad am I? I feel like ending it all, this is a bizarre life, a voice which rules my life in a way I can't make head or tail of.

Many facts are obscure, but what is clear is that the voice no longer pretends even the semblance of love and is cold towards me. I wrote a song in the bath. The voice encouraged it, but the star in his life is such that he sees no one else, knows no one else, and is so crazed with his love for her, that I can be a thread in the cotton, for all that the voice notices me. But then Miss Beyaz is very beautiful and I have never been beautiful. How I wish for some peace but there is no peace, only my desire to work and write.

Increasingly, I am isolated, because of the voice I dislike my women friends, and gay woman make me feel even more isolated, in despair and unlike the innocent girl I used to be. But then I am no longer a girl, I am a woman and a woman should not be innocent, not forever. The voice adores his new love and I can't stop him. I would not try, but there are the facts, what should I be doing while he marries, when I can not do anything without the voice? He says he'll serve me forever; all I have to do is go out with a woman. Men are cruel. He took all my lovers away, and now he does not want me. He took them away and does not feel anything, but looks at me with his cold cruel eyes, and I am fed up. I see him occasionally delivering things, and being a nuisance to his employees. I wish I knew if I was insane or not. I don't want to have women. I don't like lesbians, and I don't think they are women at all; they are different to all the women. I wish he would go away.

15-04-03

Two MacDonald's got bombed and I think Jim owns them. The last time it was Harrods and he sold it, so Jim says. I am a lunatic and my life is taking a turn. The voice offered me two billion dollars not to publish this diary. Do voices have pounds, shillings and pence?

Today has been uneventful, we went shopping with mum. We got a cotton shirt for uncle, mum's brother. I chose it and helped with the wrapping, mum doesn't know the address so I wrote it out, and then I did a booklet for the art class. Or rather I did both at the same time. All day a deep oppression of my soul gripped me and I had a scowl on my face. I keep on noticing how old I am. That is because of the voice. He keeps on comparing me with his new love, Miss Beyaz. I feel like an over weight old bag and I have started eating more; chocolates and biscuits, we had a magnum today and everything. We also went to a MacDonald's, had something to eat, luckily no bombs. Jim did not appear so all went right.

I sometimes think I am mad. I must be imagining all kinds of things about celebrities. Not that I am particularly star struck. I know too much about the hard work the stars put in. So why is my fantasy about stars? I don't know, but I am glad that the MacDonald's got bombed, so there. MacDonald's stands for greed, and power hungry slobs, that some people like to be. MacDonald's stands for the man I lost, so I am glad, but feel sad too, because I don't envy anyone who works for MacDonald's.

16-04-03

For awhile I thought of myself as a whole person, alive in every pore. But tonight I saw Miss Beyaz, her hair dyed blonde, and the voice crazy about her. I think that she is affected, but if I had the looks and the figure I would be too. Our local supermarket, that the voice purports to own, is up for sale. Kwik Save too. But I saw someone with my malady, and she had a male voice inside her, and she, poor woman, was banging her head against the wall, every so often, listening to the male voice, and banging her head against the wall. I'm trying to externalise it, aren't I? But sometimes I can swear that the voice is real. I can form sentences that he is real, but I saw a creature banging her head against the wall, because I know what the voices say to one.

They are saying become a man, they are killing me youngish. They are being awful and mean, and the voices are there with their imaginary prowess. So am I sane or insane? I don't know, if it were telepathy couldn't the man have come? I feel his kiss or rather felt his kiss, he is at the moment in love with Miss Beyaz, and he doesn't see anything or anyone except her.

Becoming a frump is what I am. The voice has become dissatisfied with me. All those years he fancied other women, he had other women and the poor mite loved only himself. Now the voice loves her and never me, and I am jealous, except when I think of that poor woman banging her head against the wall. For these couple of days I felt like that too. I felt like killing myself or being in a jail, and the lack of sex is driving me crazy, but the voice don't want to be fucked by men, and I don't want to be fucked by women. So I go without, with a bowed head, I must face my destiny of being a schizophrenic. I hate this illness, it is like nothing at all that I have experienced, it is always there tormenting me.

I can't go any further in my career but I must push myself. Today mother said that Ziynet rang and they talked. My sister and Jeanette Ju Pierre met on the train and they had words. I dislike my sister and that woman talking. Jeannette is a former friend who said she fancied me. Nothing happened, but for the voice it was a God send, he would encourage me to visit her house, and when I was attacked she came over with John, who wanted to kiss me. John is seventy years old and Jeannette is a woman. So I left that group of people, although my poetry suffered in consequence. The Meeting House was an excellent show case for my talent. I got attacked about eight years ago, or maybe more. I had my period, and was busily trying to sell my father's bracelet, when a black man relieved me of it, by stabbing me in three places. The voice would not help me identify the man. I realized then how alone I was and quit working in the cafe. There was blood everywhere and I was alone. How alone? I am very alone. The voice is just a voice, fancying blondes all over the place.

I have got to realize that I am alone. I have to go to university, but I haven't heard, and that is what is driving me nuts with despair. My sisters are more successful than I. I am not jealous any more, but I feel I must have a certain success otherwise I'll go mad. Sometimes I have cramps in my sides where I had been knifed. My face looks awful, I am looking downright vulgar. Today dad was unwell. Dad has cancer and he is not being operated on. I tried to phone the hospital but no answer. All those sick people, and father not a penny to his name. We'll die of poverty.

The voice is called Albert something, a Prince. He is the Prince of Somewhere. But if he were real, would he be so much like a voice telling me to become a man? Reading the papers about his parents I don't see the same person. Prince Albert is a virtuous youngish man. True, he never married, but maybe he did not find the perfect person.

18-04-03

I just found myself reading the business pages of the Guardian. Somerfield is worth a lot of money, 150 Somerfields, I think, for 500,000,000. That is half a billion. I think men are so precious with their businesses. Women leave to have babies but men pursue it. The voice is the owner of Somerfield, or purports to be, so I am reading all I can to find out.

My over active brain will kill me, but it is fun just reading about money. I never had any money to scratch myself with, and suddenly the voice is screaming at me not to write in my diary about him. He thinks he is this rich person with a destiny, with Miss Beyaz. But even if he were, a man does not wait six years to be married, not unless he is a prime fool. But there was publicity on TV because this star wants to marry at thirty. Beware logic in the age of modernism, that's what is killing romance. I just want to see them married so that I can have some peace. I was unfaithful to the voice, and the voice was unfaithful back. But now he is in love, and he is spoiling his love so that she can have a career. He'll be fifty in six years time. Does he think he'll live forever?

Mother saved the dog from being strangled. I called and it came, bless my dog, I love her so. Shirin slept, the old lady sleeps a lot, every time she got up she licked me, and went to sleep again. By the way, father is sleeping a lot. Uncle rang, not the one who died, but mother's brother, to say thank you for the shirt.

I just wonder if I am going mad again. Today was a sunny day, but the weather man reckon we are going to have snow. We certainly had wind. Dad was sleeping and I went to buy some ice cream, the door was open and Ataturk's picture went flying to the ground. The gust of wind had done it. I interviewed mother and framed some pictures. But it was the voice that framed them. He did it so quick I was surprised. But then, I got really tired, I had to cut the card and stick it alongside, and then stick the pictures and make a book. I like it. The voice reckons that is the best in the bunch.

If the voice is Prince, then I have to see if Prince marries Miss Beyaz, if he does, then what? I don't know, but God I wish he was kind and less insane with his own self.

19-04-03

I got up and felt the door flap go. I was so depressed, listless, that I nearly turned over and slept. Mum began reading the names on the envelopes. I rushed downstairs to see if she had read them correctly. Then I went mad with joy, I have got accepted on a BA Fine Art Course. I read and reread. Then Dad came over with some onions and said, "The bank is open". Getting dressed I was all fingers and thumbs, and I was so engrossed in my joy that I did not bother with the voice, and the voice did not congratulate me, like he always politely does, which I think is the honest feeling. Anyway I filled in the acceptance form, and was off at a trot to go to the bank and to post the letter. An unconditional offer one does not get every day. I missed one bus, and then posted the letter with feelings of relief.

Got on the bus and was at the bank. I showed them my slip of paper and they photocopied it. They did not take my finger prints, but almost. They did not give me the money. Dad has put our money into somebody else's account. All day I have felt such joyful happiness. As I walked the dog I felt happy as I read T.S. Eliot's The Wasteland, I felt happy. You know about fifteen years ago I did not understand him, but now, it is a measure of different voices, some of them female. All talking, that is the point.

I phoned my sisters and we are going to have a party tomorrow, then I rang poor Flora and she has at last sussed out what is wrong with her. Heart murmur, that is why she is feeling so tired. We talked about the university and how I could have my plays acted, maybe. I want that, but I want professional acting, and this will mean amateur theatricals. Anyway we stayed talking and she did not mention her son, except her health. I find that puzzling, maybe she was hiding something? Who knows, I wish she was telling me everything about the reason she is ill. She has been ill for ten years and not been diagnosed, they think she is potty. I completely agree, but she is sane too.

Then I had to ring off, because I told her what dad had done, dad is going to have an operation next Monday if all goes well. I also rang Aydin. I did a dreadful thing as usual with Aydin, I did not go to teach, but opted for commercial enterprise, and that came to nothing, I would have preferred teaching, at least I would have got expenses. But I did had my work displayed and sold two books. The rest just went.

Anyway I am a happy bunny. I will complete the course this time, even if I don't pass with a first class degree, I will get by.

20-04-03

Today sister is staying with us. Ziynet came bustling and happy, and we had a show case kind of a day. She read and saw my work in the Big Issue, and we were happy. Except now I have a headache due to the excitement. I walked the dog, and was happy with her until she growled at another dog. I must teach her not to. Dad is thoughtful; I think he is thinking about cigarettes. We saw Anne Frank's diary on television and I was interested. Poor Anne Frank, so much a teenager cooped up in that one flat, and then she died, but we have not got to that yet, I know what

53

will happen to her, and told it to my sister who said I spoilt the surprise.

Belgin got assaulted again. She was walking when some kids knocked her book, and made her fall. I got in when she began to scream at them saying she knew their faces. She seems all right but I don't like it, it is roughening her. That delicate girl is beginning to roughen. I am going to buy a dye to colour my hair. Belgin and me are going to Prague, Roger too will be coming, and we are going to be happy, but why does she have all those bad things happen to her? I forgot which of her stories I had read. I feel ever so guilty because she writes these bizarre stories; I don't know who will read them. Maybe some day she will be a famous authoress, but I don't think so. Her poetry, I think, is better, but she is not a serious writer. Somehow I think she will make it because she always does. No matter what she does she makes a go at it, except for writing. Is it my imagination that she has roughened? She doesn't wear make up, and she is 38 or nearly. A difficult time for a woman, but she seems to be bearing up pretty well.

The voice is still taunting me about how many lovers he's had, and how wonderful his new lover is. But who cares about the voice.

22-04-03

Today, I sent the booklet that I was working on yesterday. I must have spent hours working on it. I sent it off to a printer out of my own pocket, it will be done because the money that I'd won, I want to use to promote the Big Issue book. I am quite pleased with my efforts but don't know how many mistakes there are. Poetry Monthly press is both a vanity thing and a printer. I don't know how much vanity, how much publisher, and don't care. If I wait for editors they'll never print my stuff, and I will languish in hell for the rest of my life.

I want to have a child, but knowing the voice, it is impossible. He hates me and I don't know what to do for the best. Miss Beyaz and he keep on getting into arguments, and I think this time it is serious, but if he isn't real, then it can't be serious, can it?

I am well and truly trapped, aren't I? I can feel his breath on me but it is my breath, and I mustn't be silly, he'll never notice me because he made me into a dishwasher, and said your hands aren't spoilt yet. I am a jerk for thinking I love someone like that. I have no soul, yet I worship him and realize that part of the problem is myself. I am at fault, every time we are happy I want to flirt with somebody else. He keeps me permanently unhappy for me not to flirt. I'm sure if we went to a doctor he could fix me, but I am tired of doctors, I want to rest.

Friday is a busy day, I go to the British Museum to paint, and be with my homeless friends. Jennifer spoke to me today about what I wanted to do, now that I will be going to a university, I said I wanted the exhibition, and it will probably work out all right. I did the shopping and the syringes, all thirty of them. I did a bit of reading; I like Popcorn but dislike The Side Of Eden by Ben Elton. I have been reading poetry and such, and I feel very happy if not content

23-04-03

Today, as I waited for the train, having come from a meeting at the Big Issue, something strange happened. I discovered God again, and with that I rediscovered myself and my former arrogance. Immediately I wanted to help the world, and use the voice to help people. But the voice does not listen to me and does not want to, he wants Miss Beyaz. My faith knocked, but determined, I began to lecture on the starving millions, and the voice so comfortable with me. He agreed he has to do something to help the Africans, and the corrupt nations, which are the whites. Millions of people die each year because of lack of drugs for aids sufferers. Drug companies have hired first rate lawyers to beat them. Then I caved in. What can I do? I want to help but what can I do?

The experience of finding myself through God left me stronger mentally. I grew wings of despotism. I grew less afraid and as I painted I received my reward in 4 good pictures. Through being good one can achieve so much in art. Through personal development one gains a mastery over emotions.

What kind of experience was it? The trains began to assume a demonic atmosphere and grew less inviting. It was as if I was a voyager looking on and no one spoke to me, but I knew I had to speak to God again or never speak about anything. So I spoke, was it Satan? Was it love? I haven't prayed in eight years ever since my attack. I was knifed and lost my faith, now I travel in a no man's zone without a proper partner. The trains assumed a fat stance, and I grew terrified that the trains might turn into elephants, the voice spoke, prodded me. Anyway something did, and then my heart sort of rested, breathed. I knew exactly what I had to do. I had to persuade all those rich people to give money to save Africa. Today we have decided to give a hundred pounds to the education fund in Turkey. Where, apparently there is a shortage of teachers and space. 100 to one classes, and the teacher does not know the names of the students until end of term. Then I wanted to do much more. After I graduate I want to teach, maybe voluntarily, or maybe have children, but I think that is a dream, because there are 14 and a half million children in Turkey of school age. All desperately searching for something, all my people, and they are searching for something. I thought Africa's needs were more, but what are needs? Everything must be judged. I want to help both countries. Both

Turkey and Africa, where would I get the man to do all that? A rich man?

I go to bed. I wonder why I have such bad relationship with men and the answer is obvious, my father is such a stupid fellow, I asked him if he wanted tea and he did not like the way I asked that question, and said no he did not want a drink. He went and made it himself. He said he did not like my attitude, nor the way I asked the question, so I told dad I did not owe him anything, and I did not like his attitude. Just because I never married does not mean he can roughshod me about. But I ended up shaking and in a dither. I don't want to go to hospital again. I know those rows, they always end with me trying to take him to hospital and ending up there myself. If it was not for mother he would have been certified years ago. Mum pretends not to notice how hateful the old man is. He is going to hospital on Sunday and I must make allowances, maybe he is afraid of death.

Going back to why men treat me badly, I think I invite them to kick me, I must have a sign up my ass saying kick me. Anyway, I am going to The British Museum tomorrow, and I must rest.

24-04-03

Today I went to the British Museum after carrying my dog, because she did not have a collar I could not risk the traffic. In the museum I started to cut the mosaics, well no, not exactly, before I began to cut the mosaics I went with the group round the museum and saw some slides. It went all right. Then I started to do my own, I had nearly finished and then I thought I would do some drawings from Frieda's book. The voice, being the voice, made insinuating gestures about the hands, the bums and the tits.

Then Miss Beyaz, the voice's love, was involved in a scandal, the light of his eyes, and her star quite put out, poor thing, she has to work harder now to beat that. The voice said any more praying and ruining my day and I won't be answerable to the consequences. Apparently Miss Beyaz has a powerful lover, mum does not know who. They all say he is powerful and does not leave her side. It must be Prince Albert.

Mum's leg was aching her. and I was put out by the voice calling me names, and saying how much he loves Miss Beyaz. A man made an indecent proposal to me today, but with the voice what hope would we have? What hope do I have with anyone?

25-04-03

Today I went and had my injection, which was like a breath of cold air onto me. Dupsy was concerned that I was in such a pressure cooker situation. But she did not know the half of it, or even the quarter.

Then I went to the British Museum class and tried to clean the stone. I spent from 11 30 to 4.30 and I could not get the gouge off. I got most of it all right but not enough to make it sparkle. My hand began aching. Bill started to be flirtatious and then the voice became active with rage. I had given Bill some Vaseline and the voice did not like it. Then, when I went on the train I tried to lick my hand, the voice's rage could not be stopped. He was as if changed from the gentleman, and became insane with loathing, and, dare I say? Jealousy.

I don't understand it. I don't understand how one part of my brain can be so much enraged like a man. Anyway I tried to calm it down, but it would not, it was jealous, and I knew if I did not do anything he would do something drastic. So I began to read the paper. Was I scared? No, father used to do that to mother, but now I am doing the raging, and everything else all by myself.

Miss Beyaz has a new hairstyle and she really does look beautiful, almost as beautiful as she would like to be.

Jennifer sent off the application form. I hope we get the award. Pam rang about a publisher. I had news that they are looking for mad people to write for them. I fit the bill, I am good and mad. I'll probably have to work at being published. Apparently the publisher finds sponsors and they publish one's work. I am so pleased I will be able to join the mainstream publications. Tomorrow is Saturday, or rather it is already, and the night is silent with everything up for grabs. I have done a bit of drawing and painting and I feel revitalized, almost like a young woman. I feel like I am three people. There is the unconfident me, and then there is the man, and there is this other me whom the male voice loves, the confident intelligent person who has reason by her side to sooth the voice. This person has bags of energy. Last night I was controlled by this voice with a vengeance and a determination. I have been broken for years and now suddenly I am whole, and able to see so clearly. It is as if this woman that I sometimes become, can do everything so well, as if she has grace, as if she is somebody else, and I am afraid of her. All my life I have been hiding from this man. This hated Erturk, the child abuser, and if he had seen me he would have killed me, despite being terrified of going to prison. He would have broken my being. So I hid. But I hid too well. I hid so well I lost myself and no one could love me.

Ziynet rang, her cat was put down and I worry about Shirin. That old cat, always in fights about territory, am I going to be like that too after growing old? I think so, men always like being fought over.

26-04-03

Talking about territory, Pamela Stephenson, the voices ex, kept him more content and happy than when he is with Miss Beyaz. Am I living in a dream world? In other words am I fantasizing this man? (Mum says that I don't talk, that I am letting them do all the things, like run a house. I was reading the papers today. What I have retained I like, but one never retains all that one reads, if I see something I can connect to, but I never remember things, it is as if my mind has become dead. That enquiring mind as a child which I had has become clouded over, like a mish mash of dreams that has escaped my grasp.

I am so jealous that it is nobody's business. I feel like screaming in sexual agony and frustration. But there is always a tomorrow, and today can be as sad as anything, then a rainbow peeps, the sun comes out, and everything is made all right.

Tomorrow dad is going into hospital; we have to wait for the phone to ring confirming a bed. But the NHS, apparently, is going down hill with the wastage of human life and people waiting endlessly to be operated on. Dad has been waiting for two months. Today he complained of being tired out. Ziynet rang about wanting a car. That Ziynet! There is always a something. Then Roger rang about me sharing a bed with a total stranger. I have not been able to say no, after all I am not paying for it, and so I must do as am told.

But I am not best pleased. After all I am a sick woman, and who knows what kind of a person the woman is?

Somebody is hooting their car; I have not heard that in years. The voice is reading this and all seems okay. I have looked at the booklet I am doing and finally I have proofread it. It is almost ready to go to print. It doesn't mean a thing. I'll give it to a few places where hopefully I'll be reviewed, and may be it will sell. If it does not, then I have been out of pocket for 70 pounds only, and I can afford that, just about.

Soon university will begin, and soon my foundation year will end, and I will be able to do things like have more money. Soon my life will be a life worth living instead of jerking round the voice and thinking when he'll have the strength to ditch or kill me. Soon my life will have more meaning, but I will never be well, schizophrenia is a disease which affects one in a hundred, is it? That is a lot of people talking to themselves like crazy, same here.

27-04-03

I got out of bed the wrong way today; I was so careworn and pale. My moon face was pinched and white and I showed my years. Dad has not been admitted due to lack of beds. He is going to have the operation tomorrow. How? The logic escapes me. He will be starved at home, and it is nearly twelve, and he shouldn't eat a thing. Tomorrow at seven a mini cab will come to pick him up with us, and then we will go to the hospital. I told them he is a diabetic and everything, and if it was not for Ziynet he would be still waiting. Ziynet rang the hospital and became bossy, said they should admit him. Before that, I nearly cancelled my holiday, in fact I did cancel it, but Roger, luckily, will wait until tomorrow. So tomorrow we will go to the hospital, and hopefully dad does not eat tonight, tomorrow is the day. God help us.

I have been painting away, I wrote a poem on Africa, and now the book is like I want it. Hopefully, I can send it off tomorrow. On the radio I heard bits and pieces of Congreve, I like him, but it was not until the end that I knew what the plot had been. I liked the end of the play, there were such depths of feeling and language in the piece, and such tremendous vim about the male female situation. I would not mind hearing it again, which I will probably, because I was sleeping most of the time, or I was on the phone. The wit reminded me of Oscar Wilde.

I must get going on a play, but I have dried up and can't write a play, all my avenues have been explored; I am finished as a playwright. I need a new subject. I haven't finished any book that I might adapt. Oh, how lazy am I?

The voice in my head is still going strong. The voice's new love is content, a woman of the world and a beauty into the bargain, so they are all satisfied with each other, and with the world. It is like watching pigs with snotty noises going huff. The pretentiousness of being pretentious is more than I can bear. I am seriously thinking of evacuating this body and going some place else. This body is mine but the poor man is castrating me. I was so overpowered today that I slept and slept, but then I woke and tried to work on something. I'm afraid of going mad again. If I go mad again I think I will end it all, for I won't go through it all again.

I don't know how much longer I can watch her flaunting herself in front of me, and smirking, she is actually smacking her lips and smirking, and because she is beautiful, the men love her and the women congratulate her. Some of them are tearing their hair, true, but that is because of the former lovers of this man.

29-04-03

Yesterday father had the operation on his cancer. I went twice to see him but he appeared well. Today, he was discharged and mother is nursing him. I am trying desperately to sooth mother and the dog. I took the dog out twice for a walk. Dad could not walk near me, he nearly fell down. Susie is feeling frustrated. They gave dad a tablet to get rid of the germs, and when I heard, that, for awhile they are infectious, anyone using the toilet could get it, I felt fear, and a shying away as if a part of dad has died.

But I am all right now. Ziynet took dad and mum away from the hospital, she helped discharge him. She basically interpreted and did what I normally do. I am ever so grateful to her, and I went to class, three of them, one after another, first sculpture and then making a book of your own, and then art theory. I need to buy a notepad and carry it with me.

When I heard, after phoning mum, that dad was home, I was amazed. But it is better that they discharge him, because with dad's lack of sanity he would have gone mad in there.

Miss Beyaz had her big night, she mumbled into the microphone and had a round of applause, and made believe that she was thirty instead of 23. You know if it was not for the voice I would feel sorry for her. She has no vocal ability to speak of, I think she should have the operation to make her sound better. Anyway, the voice is depressed because his pet has been found wanting, and this rich guy whoever he is, the lover who I think is Alfred, is to blame. Why should a perfectly unspoilt, untalented, little housewife material be made into a laughing stock? She fares better as an actress, but she pretends to be dignified and older which takes away from the enjoyment. She is affected. I must rest.

Today I had good news, they like my Frieda Kahlo impressions, and they said that one day it will be published. They reckon it is the best thing I have done, but editors and classroom critics always say that. I work hard and never amount to anything.

Leyla my friend was crying today, and when I went to sit by her table she said she did not get into university. She had applied to St Martin's and she did not get in. John Sheehy did not know that he had to sign the acceptance form, so he photocopied the UCCAS form and put it on the mantelpiece. When I told him he was surprised, he was very bemused. I have been applying for grants left, right, and centre. The house needs to be oiled with money, otherwise I would not be able to go to university. The cafe makes 500 a month profit but never stretches far enough. There is always a hole, always a new demand on mother, and the finances don't perk beyond a couple of thousand, and we seem always to be in debt.

I walked the dog and now she is barking. It is nearly twelve thirty and my eyes are black with shadows, the dog is barking and father can't find his pyjama top. I found it for him, and now we all can go to bed and sleep the exhausted sleep of the just.

30-04-03

Today I had an easy work schedule. I went to the Big Issue and ran a writing class, but we did not agree on the Radio programme we were going to do. I rang the radio station, left a message and then went looking for another copy of the Big Issue. Then we were chucked out of the room, someone else wanted to use it. Sometimes I think I am going to commit suicide. Not because of work, but because of the cruel voices.

This voice in my head is saying such beastly things to me. It is saying it loves Miss Beyaz, it is saying he hates me, it is saying he doesn't want anything to do with me, and he adores this other woman. It is saying that this other woman does not fart in public and I do. It is saying he doesn't want me. Well and good, but what if everybody was schizophrenic, then I think it would be hell for everyone, and we can jolly well have an all night party.

The voices in my head have been active and I don't want to bloody know. The voices keep on at me even when I am reading the newspaper. What botheration why can't I be a normal woman and not hear them? Mum says that it is in my hands, if I was stronger maybe they would go away. But I am beginning to look my age, I am nearly forty four and still hear the Goddamn voice.

People who don't have to live with schizophrenia are the luckiest people in the world. For not one moment is ones own, the greatest crime is to be schizophrenic, and it is awful. I hate the voice and the voice hates me, but we still find loads of things in common, like we both have shops we think need us. Lloyds, which is my bank, has cut down staff in what the Guardian reports is panic selling. One in three staff is gone.

The voice also wants to invest in Turkey, a bit more risky there, for they make their fortunes very quickly and lose it with equal rapidity. It is always so. There are so many corrupt individuals there. Anyway, one must not stand in the way of young love. The voice and Miss Beyaz have cooked themselves in a holy passion, both making money, and both having a fair degree of sex. That is what is so strange, maybe these people are real. At least Miss Beyaz I know is real, but the man has always been a shadowy thing, distantly remembered.

Dad is better. We went and bought a hoover, because mum refuses to clean the carpets with the brush. So we bought a carpet cleaner which sucks the water. It is coming tomorrow and I am going to classes. Mum and I are going to collect the rent.

1-5-03

We went and collected the rent, and then I went and tried to draw. First, I took Susie out and we had a nice walk. I just love walking with Susie, I seem to be busy all the time. I did not read the paper all that much, only to the international pages, because I fell asleep. I slept from 8 till midnight, so it is, in reality, the 2nd of May, but I am writing about yesterday, and that is what counts. Spoke to the tenant and he said his wife has breast cancer. Did not dare mention that dad has cancer, or had it. But Joe seemed to be relishing in his bad fortune. He said he would have preferred it if her breast had been removed. Then she would not be in danger, she has apparently had chemotherapy, I told him my good news about getting into university, he was expecting something like it, and appeared relieved. I think he is relieved that we would be too busy to put the rent up.

The voices were not so beastly today, and I enjoyed a relative quietness I don't enjoy normally. The hoover came, mum doesn't think it is a good machine, "I wish I had bought the one in the catalogue." This is quite good I told her, it is what everyone uses, but she did not think so, then we put it together and she still could not agree; now we are waiting for Belgin to fix it, because I can't for the life of me make it work. I am not the most mechanical person.

I went to drawing class, told everyone my good news, and then I went to my writing class, did the rounds with the good news, but 'a well fed man's table is different from a famished man's table'. They laughed, though some, dare I say, were pleased that I was leaving. Then Kerry read her piece and it was stunning, it was excellent, if only I could get the atmosphere so right, the words so succinct. If only I could write better. Then it was

Joan's turn and it was not as good, but good in its way. I enrolled for the poetry class, after enrolling for my creative writing course. But if I am to go to Prague I won't be able to go for a week, and that I think will be terrible. I wish I could get Big Issue people more interested in writing, these people are top brains, and we at the Big Issue writing group are disadvantaged. All the best brains are not coming, and do their work behind the scenes. I want the Big Issue people to have the best possible things. I tried yesterday, but they oversleep and come half way through the writing class, they are desperate to make money and in writing there is only work, not money!

2-05-03

Today has been a mixture of sorts, with the voice shouting out his love for Miss Beyaz and being really abusive. I looked like an old hag and felt like one too. Then I met this delicious person called William. He is in his early thirties and he wants to do art. He also wants to become an English teacher. I like him. He reminds me of Ted and he seems to like me, which is strange and unfamiliar. It has been a long time since anyone liked me.

But the voice is objecting, how am I going to go to bed with him when he could see us naked together? Well I don't give a damn, he has his Miss Beyaz and I will have my William. It is so boring being in a threesome when I am the discarded tampon. You know all that writing I had done about Turkish men, well the voice played it upon me. He neglected me, he cuckolded me, and now I think it is time he went elsewhere and did his cuckolding. I am fed up to the teeth with the voice, what has he done recently but abuse me?

William is quite young and looks even younger. The voice is bringing images of his Miss Beyaz. You know I see her on the television smirking, and I see her in my minds eye, and she is smirking. She is smirking just like Pamela Stephenson, and I just want to be ordinary, and have a life, not with the crumbs, but with my own sanity, and as a woman. No one can make me become a lesbian, and no one can make me kill myself through abusive behavior.

I met William at the Printing class and he seems interested in me. We had a nice discussion about the printmaking which the teacher exhibited. We seem to be polite strangers at the moment, and William did say he has a girl friend but ... I know, I know I'll be hurt, but who cares what will happen? I want to be hurt by somebody else.

I am reading Conrad at the moment, and I think he was a racist but in a good natured way. He does have a scene about cannibals, and how unappetizing the natives must see him, because apparently natives do nothing but eat people. Maybe it was the mentality of those people at that particular time, but I like the strong writing even though every other sentence one can't agree with. I read bits of it to a black woman called Nanna, who is recently married, and she seemed to be good natured, but for life of me the more I said about the book the more quiet she grew.

No, Conrad was not writing for black people, he was writing for the middle classes, the male white something. It is all something these days, thirty something, twenty something, forty something.

I did a couple of prints which weren't bad, but it was not as intensive as I would have liked them to be. And I am not tired, I am faintly tired like something dreamy and calm, and I know the voice will try it on, but no, he is involved with Miss Beyaz. He gave Pamela, according to the voice, 37,000,000 pounds just to keep quiet about his affair with her. I wonder if that is real or if I am making it up?

As Conrad said we all make up some things. The voice is a pathological liar. In fact he is insanely jealous of his privacy. He doesn't like this diary.

3-05-03

I had a really enlightening day. I went to a tutorial and then we all talked about the exhibition we are going to have. June 21 it would be, and it is called the longest day. I voted for something completely different. One of my friends has had a by-pass done to him, and he said that he has run out of time. I had today loads of peanuts and my heart does not feel very well, but I have oceans of time, I guess.

Today he voice doesn't want me to be with William, and it has been so tender and loving that it's nobody's business. It has turned my head into a stable. I am fed up about the voice, and if I had my life over again I would not even condescend to listen to it.

Then I listened to the radio about what is self? And I wonder if I have a self? Or am I going round and round in circles? The voice is making funny faces and trying to make me laugh, but it is no good, the essence of self is goading me on. Why do schizophrenics listen to their demons and the rest of the population don't? Mum does say that everyone has a voice in their heads, so what makes me a dual personality and not mother?

I know that I am sick but how sick I don't know. The voice can go and hang itself.
It is as if I am still being abused. It is as if I am in the receiving end of all that is bad, and it is the voice that is doing it. I am repeating what Halil did, and the voice is supplying the torture in this torturous world. I sometimes want to pack it in and go to Cyprus where one can live with the world on top of one. I am really bad tonight for I think that

my ex is having sex with someone else, and it is driving me insane with jealousy.

Why can't I accept that it is over and done with? Why must I punish myself? But as the years pass my feelings are as strong as ever, and as I put the light out to go to sleep I am feeling my way towards a light, and the light is not there, it is a reflection. I push and shove to be a writer but I am clumsy, and my fear is people will notice my clumsiness is there, warning me that I am not a genius, that my talent is in my superficiality and envy towards others. I wonder if this line makes sense. As the days go and I am locked in this battle I am not even strong enough to bear it. I am not strong but I am a woman. Read the notices of death today in the Guardian and found something which I completely agreed with. Those women who have sex with women are not women. What are they? The feminist have gathered strengths and have made something of the rights of women, but in Turkey women are treated far worse than here in this civilised country, how many women suffer too but, because it is their choice, are silent.

5-5-03

It will be Belgin's birthday soon. Men are all alike; every man that I have ever met wanted to know what I think. Is that the reason I've become schizophrenic? My hair is a mess! My life is a mess. I am a mess. I saw Miss Beyaz on Turkish television. She seems to be coping well with being a star. The voice in my head wants to marry her. I wake up at night dreaming that I have married her. Then wake and blissfully I am alone. This is good, to be alone is good. I guess everybody is alone. We all sleep alone. I have had voices in my head for most of my life and I am tired of it. My voices have made me gullible. A terrible innocence in my youth was beset with poverty. When one has money one is not innocent for long, for they come at you and destroy it, but when one is poor they leave you to wallow in your innocence. I was neither beautiful or sexy so they left me alone.

Dad's cancer is not cured. He has to have chemotherapy. The letter came on Saturday; I put it to one side without reading it properly because I had to be at College. Life bustling, life forever sucking one until there is endless momentum. I just read one appointment. How the hell was I to read all the rest when I was so busy? So 24 hours later my sister comes, we have lunch at a restaurant, the one we always go to. We talk, laugh, and the kids there, and dad as white as a sheet. Mother beside herself with joy because she is seated next to her grand daughter. We are so happy, not a care in the whole wide world. Then we realize how poor we've become, how destitute. Is father dying? The doctors are so clumsy with machines, that they don't work, and his cancer growing.

I must be mad, life is not for me, and the relentless life moves me. Black grapes are good for cancer, and tomatoes, carrots and fish. Dad is glum, he looks ready for death. Death prepares him. We don't have much time. He sits listening to the news gloomily. But I could die before he does. I know I could disagree with the voice and jump in front of the train. But it could have been much worse, our children could have had it, like the neighbours. Or mother, but mother sits and rests her leg, and then she jumps up making tea and doing the gardening, or washing the dog, or just cleaning the carpets. She doesn't want to be creative, saying her home is her creation. I row with the voice endlessly, and the quarrelsome chap does nothing but make eyes at every women. I sense that now we are at a crossroads. I just want to die.

The editors won't give me money. I work hard but there is no market for what I am doing. I am an empty vessel whose life is nothing but a burden. The voice is insisting that I become a lesbian, and yet more rows. I said he could marry whoever he likes. I am tired of the argument. Do you know Miss Beyaz was fat as a teenager? So she did not eat, and now has advanced vitamin deficiency, this has caused her to be forgetful and she can't have children.

A thing of beauty lasts forever, except for women. No, a woman has until she is forty for her physical beauty to fade. Then it is all downhill. I don't feel well. The house is quiet as if someone is about to snuff it, all asleep. Even the dog has quietened down. All the clocks are fast, too fast. I worry about everything.

6-05-03

Nearly half a year has passed. I have to have my injection and my cholesterol pills. I haven't had them for a couple of days. I feel heavy and sluggish. I went to college today, 10.30 till 8P.M, non stop. I painted some images and it was fun. I had a tutorial, we talked about Charlotte Salome and how young she was killed. Salome had been twenty six and pregnant and was shot by the Nazis. Then I studied art in a capital manner. I will be in college on Friday and Tuesday, and then I go on holiday. I put on my summer dress; it was cold to begin with. My pen is running dry, but I am gaining confidence as men looked, not women. When I feel ugly it is women who look, they pity me. When I feel pretty, men look. Today I felt like that and a man came and tried it on. The voice stepped on his toes. I raced away, if the man had quarrelled with me what would I have said and done? I don't like anyone coming near me anymore, men and women are taboo.

8-05-03

Today I did things, like the book is coming along. The pamphlets I sold, or gave away. I still feel sluggish. I am bankrupt. I must get some money from some place. Our Prime Minister is 50.

The world comes roses for him. He has done something with his life. I might be on the radio, amateur radio. I spoke to a woman and she seemed interested. So we will go as a group. I will be busy tomorrow. Today I slept in class, I couldn't believe it. Kerry wouldn't buy my book. Well rich people don't, and Kerry is very rich. She is the one who brought a fantastically good piece about this Nazi concentration camp.

Guilt in my heart, but I've done nothing to be ashamed of. They are demons in my head. I know no peace, which is killing me. If only there was peace. So days pass in hell. My hell began twenty years ago and there is no end to my suffering.

He loves somebody else and where do I go? The same body, different heads. He loves somebody else and I am one too many. You see my hell has no respite. I eat and sleep. I bought a book by Wanda Barford, read it on the bus. It is lovely, all about her beautiful mother. Her mother was like a child who said she can't be bothered and went to tea with her sister, and poor Wanda telephoned all over, then, when she phoned the right house, her mother without a trace of guilt called her darling, I can't be bothered. My mum never did that, except when she was not able due to illness, due to violence from dad. Dad did lock me out once while he went out, and I had to sleep with a boy who kicked. Wanda did not buy my book.

9-05-03

Belgin is 38 today and we phoned her first thing in the morning to congratulate her. Actually Belgin only gets cross when she is trying to fix my computer. I've not bought her a present, not because I am mean but because I don't have any money. The pamphlet ate away my money.

Today I went to the Big Issue and scanned some images and became a writer instead of an artist. Stayed from 11.30 till about 4.30 editing the book. I liked Jason Dore's work very much indeed, but Fabini's I don't, I am going to edit her until she gets a calling card. Flora did edit me until I learnt. So I think Fabini should be edited too.. Then I went to the Print workshop and there was only me for an hour. I did a few good things, but I forget other things that she taught me. Then everyone came and did fantastic work, except me.. This must be the advanced stuff. I used the wheel and things became beautiful. Fay, the teacher, bought John the student's work, and I think they like each other. William did not come and I was not devastated.

10-05-03

The voice today was not aggressive, in fact it was sweet, there was an argument but it was so minor it blew over. I have applied for a scholarship, a thousand pounds, and the voice said that it was its claret. It is one expensive voice I have to tell to you. Whatever I earn it belittles and I end up not earning anything. It is like that about my money. I wonder if it is like that about Miss Beyaz's money? After all she is a millionairess. But the voice can go and hang itself, I am going to enjoy myself with my money, and it can talk about millions as if they grew on trees. I wonder if it is possible to kill a voice? I have been thinking about it quite seriously, but who will do the typing?

The voice does not fancy me, it fancies this other woman. Today I dressed up in my oldest rags and went out. I took my mum and dad with me and we had a good meal. Mum and Dad had an argument about smoking, dad said how good a cigarette is, and mum said it kills. Then he went out and came back but without a cigarette. Dad is like on a leash, and he will be untied, loose to roam at will. Mum has started to scrum his back, and I think there might be sex involved, but they are so old. Dad is nearly seventy, but he still enjoys mum. I am happy for them.

My printer is not working, I think it needs a clean. So I could not send off the application, and why does the voice not want me to have money? Whenever I do, it says but you'll have a lot, and I end up giving it away! Why? It is odd. It is like I am a burden on the world and I can't seem to breath.

I hope to finish reading Conrad tomorrow, and the paper, and to finish Freida Kohle pastel sketches. I am still thinking about Wanda's mother, I find it intriguing that a woman should love her mother to write a whole book on her. I hope to write one on my mother too. Dad is gaining his confidence and that is dangerous for him, he tends to bully everyone, and smoke.

11-05-03

I did a picture of a tree, I don't think that it was good. I have been sluggish. I took the dog for a walk and was in a filthy mood. So she did not enjoy the walk. I left painting, I can't seem to concentrate. I nearly forgot to pack my passport. My medicines I have now packed. But if it was not for mother, asking me if I had thought about my passport, I would have gone without it. I don't know, but every day I am more and more forgetful.

I have to do ten more sketches and then I can rest from art. I have to take "The Scream" to the college. I did a color wheel. I read the newspaper but without really going deeply into it. I am so sluggish and confused.

Why? Because in my other dimension I see glamorous people and I know them. I have no glamour myself so how can I know someone of that much stature? I don't think that telepathy is possible so why aren't I having sex with someone, anyone. But the voice is insisting that I don't have sex, not even with the voice. He used to cuddle me but now he says he is in love with someone else, and does not want to be unfaithful. I feel so frustrated that I don't think I am sane. It is worse than being in prison, for in prison there is a reprieve, a way out, but how can one go out of one's head and start again? How can days pass and nothing but work to do, nothing, but nothing to do? I am getting older and older and nothing is happening.

Am I a complete nonentity? Am I so non existent that no one can see me, and no one can know me because I am a frustrated old hag? I am old, I must admit, but to be old and never loved is the worse that can be. I am old and unloved and I want so desperately to be young and full of life and love, but I am twisted and bitter, and no one in their right minds would come to me and love me. So days pass, and years gather dust over me, and there is no one to watch over me, and no one to love me, because I am old and useless, and spots in my face as big as boils, and no one to kiss it better, and no one to make me a woman, and that is that.

I have a lot to do tomorrow and a lot to get through. I hope I remember everything important. I must phone the repair people about my computer. I also must phone about father and go to the library, and then I must get my injection, that is important, and then I must go with mother and shop, and then I must go to the bank and get some money, and then I must do a great deal of organizing. Suzy must be walked, the cat reassured, and I must send the scholarship form back, and to do that I need to get to a library.

On Tuesday I got class and I hope to work hard, and then go to my sister and stay the night, for we must make an early start. So tonight is the only rest I might be having, and tonight is already Monday morning. It is nearly one o'clock and I am feeling much better, it is as if the diary puts everything into perspective, all my sufferings I can air, and be so gently removed. I hope to have everything cleared and aired and made safe. I am a victim of the voice, and if I die, who is to know how much I have suffered, and will go on suffering, even when I am dead there won't be peace for I had a vision, and the vision said that if I commit suicide it would be hell. I can always have thoughts like that, and my sanity is something precarious that I have to fight over.

Mum dreamt of my uncle who died of cancer, she dreamt of a light, and how my uncle and his wife were together, and there was a light, and how they shut the door. I wonder if everyone in Cyprus is all right, and if the money we sent did not reach them? Is auntie all right, she took it so much to heart when uncle died, and I would not like her being dead, for who else would I go to see in Cyprus?

12-05-03

Tomorrow I am going to college and then to my sister, and on the 14th we are going on holiday. Today I was bad, really insane. A post office van nearly drove into me. It honked its horn and then I crossed the road. I could not renew my library books because the library is on strike. I went to the one in Woolwich, apparently they want better wages. I have been phoning for days and days, and the phone is answered by a machine which states the time it opens, but it is never open. I expect librarians have to live too. Do writers live? Well I barely survive.

I went and had my injection. The needle was thrust into my bum so hard it was as if a ligament had been torn, and I did not even gasp, or maybe I did, it was as if my bum was on fire, and the needle, even when he pulled it away, was in.

I am going insane but who cares, who wants to know? Days and days pass and no one turns up. Years pass, and I age and I age and I age and that is that. I am angry at it, I want to stop this but can't. And today I nearly solved it but the driver was a good driver.

Then I calmed down. I ain't a lunatic for nothing, you know. I always know the bright side. But what is a bright side? When some jerk thrusts a needle so hard at your side that they destroy the last vantage of dignity one's got? That one's illness is a part of the facts of life, and that one can't get away from it? No matter, it will be all right and I will be well. But when? When will I be well? So days pass in a stupor and I can't even write good stuff, and I can't paint, and I can't do print making without having someone showing me up as incompetent. Because I am incompetent. I am a lazy so and so who does nothing all day but try to read the paper, and then only the first few lines and the headlines.

I can't sit properly, I think my period is on its way, and I am having a night at home, mother, poor soul, is worried. I am too worried they need me, Suzie needs me, and I need them.

The voice has been very active today, and his love of Miss Beyaz is growing and growing. The voice won't let me be happy, every time I am happy he wants to know why I am happy, and why I am looking at men. He says that Miss Beyaz does not look at men, and I should be like her.
My backside hurts.

I saw a film once, and the voice reckons I am like the woman in it. You know, after everything in trousers, and so I bid myself good night.

I sent off the scholarship application, my printer is not working so I wrote it by hand.

15-05-03

We are in Prachod in the Czech Republic, or is it prats land in cuckoo land? It took us the best part of yesterday and the previous day to travel, from 2.30 to 7pm. Roger had not booked a room, and there was a delay on the rail. So we waited on the station for nearly two precious hours, and my thoughts took on a darkness. I thought we would be homeless for certain. Then in Jicin we got off the slow train and went to an information centre, we had 20 minutes to find a room. One had no windows and was cold, and the other was too expensive, Belgin and Roger still looked through the brochure. I did not want to be out in the streets. But they were serene, used to this, I thought of the extremes of the situation. What if we were robbed, murdered? And, as I sat in the chair with the table in front of me, looking at the bags we had, memories of being a bag lady over came all common sense.

As I waited for them to be less touristy, desperate to save their money, I realize that we were in a predicament, it was 5.30 and the Tourist Office closed. We were in it, and the girl, who, luckily, could speak English, booked us a room. The rooms are warm, but there aren't any doors between one room, and the double room. The shower is in the double room and goes cold as one uses it, but the rooms are comfortable, with central heating warming my bones.

Yesterday's journey is still in my mind's eye. The growing nightmare of having everything on one's back, and the great outdoors, with nothing between you but your bags. The flight had been all right, we had food on the plane but when we had got to the rooms, no food, no amenities, no nothing, and I suggested we go to a hotel to see if we could find that elusive food, and we were too late, much too late, so Belgin who had ate only biscuits and was hungry, looked longingly at the food, and I who had chocolate looked sick and tired. We came out of the hotel depressed and cold.

This morning I woke up so hungry and thirsty. First thing I suggested we go and have breakfast, and we got there just on time. I walked so fast. As fast as my little legs would carry me and we were on time. We ate and we ate. We took some with us, paid 210 crowns. When we left there was hardly any food on the serving table. Breakfast over we went outside and I was happy, and the day was good It was worth every penny.

Then we climbed Cesky Prochov. I tried to walk but it was difficult, and the voice took over the walking. The voice and me hated each other, and as I walked the voice insinuated that I fancied him, and wanted to destroy his life with his Miss Beyaz.

So we walked and walked, and then it did not matter any more, it was a wash out, and now I am going to the Bistro to have some coke. We have finished our walk, at least I have. I've been twice to the Bistro, and the wood fire is not burning, and it's very shut. I am cold, and I am waiting for Belgin and Roger, because we plan on going to the hotel again to have something to eat. I have rested and now I want to talk and socialise. I haven't read the Guardian in two days, and I don't know what's been happening in the world. But seemingly the planet must be okay, because we are still here and existing.

Roger wants me to spend more of my money, but Belgin had suggested I come and she'd pay for the holiday, and now she has changed her mind. I seem to be paying all the time. Roger even suggested I pay the train fare but Belgin said it was okay. She paid, but how long?

16-05-03

We packed. Took our possessions on our backs and, without the landlord collecting the keys, we waited a bit, but couldn't wait forever. Roger did say between 8-9. We had a train to catch. So we left our room and went through grassy mud and broken bridges. Belgin's bag is so heavy, and Roger is carrying my bags.

We asked an ambler about the station and he took pity on us, showing the way. We walked three kilometres to a station. We were just on time to catch the train, but we only went one stop, and then we were on our way to Prague.

The former night we had a discussion about taxis and luckily I had lost, for the landlord might never have arrived in time. The slow train stopped at all stations as if a terrible lethargy was on it. The train stopped every 2 minutes. A woman got on with a pram. These trains are steep, it's not possible to board without injury, but the baby was sleeping as if it was as safe as a house.

After four hours, we arrived in Prague. Where, in a matter of minutes my peace was disturbed by a man asking us if we wanted accommodation. I said no and Roger said yes. On tenterhooks as they bargained. So we paid 3 nights lodging, £95. We went and had a look at the place and it seemed clean, but we are not allowed to breathe let alone live. We stay outside, there are people living in the flat. The flat had been flooded, but now it is a good, comfortable place. No visitors allowed and no loud music. Belgin, poor thing, must get her shoes off to walk. I thought, as we lost our way, after eating with Margaret, that the Metro had moved, that we would never see our bags again. My legs could not carry me further.

Who is Margaret? She is running the marathon with Roger, and I fear the voice. Miss Beyaz and the voice. I was crying last night. I snored apparently. But in the end we were safe and sound, and now I am going to bed. I wanted to end it all today but I did not. For some strange reason I go on...

18-05-03

Yesterday I ate and ate. I also went to a museum, (The National), which is a Natural museum. We walked so much, there is a MacDonald's in front of the Museum so I naturally gravitated there. I bought the Daily Mail and read. The mail cost 70 crowns but it had black lettering about Europe. I think we should join Europe, why shouldn't we? Europe I see as great, and will block American imperialism.

I was not bored my in company, and the people surrounding me formed a hollow gravity that pulled me to life as a living organism, I was interested in my surroundings. There was a mother with her kids, and there came a man with his burgers onto my table, and sat suggestively in front of me. I was not interested; I don't have sex any more. I stayed an hour killing time by reading and looking at the clock.

They came, and we left for the pasta party. After all the walking I have blisters, and as I expected, Margaret tried it on. I said nothing to my sister but suspected that she might have arranged it. It was only later that I learnt she thought nothing of the sort, that she did not know that Margaret was that way inclined, and that in fact she thought me mad. Margaret apologized and left on the bus.

I feel so old. The voice and I have nothing but arguments. I am fed up. The voice says that it does not like being written about, but that's my one consolation, writing about my daily life. Today Roger is running the marathon and so is Margaret. I got up at 7.30 and tried to be ready in time, but was late. I found Belgin alone, waiting for me on the landing. Roger had already left for the marathon. Belgin, with difficulty blew up the balloons, and Roger and Margaret passed, I don't think I like what's been in my mind. My suspicious mind. But the voice is pushing to have a female to female relationship. He will catch air.

The loud music of the marathon makes me realize how changed I am from the girl who loved things wild. I now think of nothing but food and the day that I will die. I don't like the kind of people I attract. Today I went to the Jewish quarter and had a look at the synagogues. One was stark and bare, it had small wooden benches and empty walls. It was terrible, and the graves we saw, one stacked on another. I wanted to go to the cemetery too, but it was too expensive. I had glimpses of genocide.

I had Belgin all to myself but she was distracted. We had lunch near the boats. The herds of people we left behind, and went to a quiet restaurant. I had spinach pancake and the spinach was not gritty.

Then we went to MacDonald's and I had a tea and ice cream. Belgin parked me there while she went to look for Roger. I went to the Communist Museum and I saw thousands of people imprisoned for crimes against the state, and spies, and realize that without greed mankind won't survive. It is self interest that keeps us alive. So after that, Belgin came to tell me we had waited, maybe, in the wrong MacDonald's, and she was going to the next MacDonald's. Then I went out of the museum and saw Belgin waiting for me.

She told me she had found Roger. We went to the next Mac Donald's and found Roger pale and tired. He had been sick and we bought him chocolate..

19-05-3

We got up, but I kept Belgin and Roger waiting in the corridor because I thought the meeting time was 8.15 when it was 7.45. A tiredness has come over me and I don't want to move. A tiredness I have which is akin to hopelessness and misery. We have bought tickets and are at Melnika: nothing is open. The voice and I had a terrible talk, and I think if it had been a real man one of us would have had to go.

We can't agree on anything. The same woman is between us. I can't seem to get what the voice, who happens to think he is a prince, wants. He doesn't know either. Or he wants what most of the planet wants, a woman who is youthful with sex appeal. He promised he would get me that too. Anything to keep me quiet. I said no thank you, and five minutes later we had the same row. He keeps on mentioning the party when I French kissed Angel. That was 21 years ago and I haven't kissed anyone since.

Everything is getting complicated. I don't want to kiss women. I hate lesbians. Women are friends or mothers or sisters. Not lovers. But the voice who claims to be Prince Albert of Monaco is adamant. He wants me to become a lesbian. Why? Because he wants to marry.

Life is one terrible mistake after another, a journey full of wrong destinations. Today is restful, the bus journey was uneventful. The trams were not crowded. Every one in the bus was full of purpose, they had things to do. But the day after tomorrow I'll have many things to do. It'll begin to seem like this is nothing but a distant dream.

But now it's real. It is the most real thing on the planet. I bought presents. I will make a good Santa. Ziynet's birthday is this week. I'm grateful to my sister because she's got kids, and she allows me to look after them. I bought the kids dolls, and Leyla an expensive doll. I hope she likes it. I bought Ted and Ziynet a face handmade.

I bought mum a tablecloth and some sort of another tablecloth, but less expensive.

I don't know what to buy dad, clothes not too cheap. So I am not buying him anything.

20-05-03

Last day today, and yesterday's inspiration is today's work. I have an idea for a play which excites me. I'm going to call it Charles Bridge and its all about the saints.

Belgin, opposite me, is eating cheese omelette, and Roger is beside her, and he has just finished his salad. I am rather the worse for wear. I feel like someone has bashed a hole in me. I went to a museum and saw a typical pre revolutionary kitchen. Black walls, because the cooking was done on a metal shelf, coal and twigs.

We went to St Barbara and I slept on the grass for ten minutes. I was refreshed and got up. But I was wearing a wrap round skirt and I showed a bit of leg. Kutna Hora is so poor everyone wants your money.

We went to a poor soup kitchen and I ate two soups, two breads and had a nice cup of tea. There were no seats and one stood and ate. The voice is vile and horrible; I wish I could get rid of it. But if I do get rid of it, I risk being a mental retard. I don't want to be handicapped.

21-05-03

It's two o'clock in the morning and I am all packed, ready to go. I've got 20 pounds left. I changed a tenner yesterday and Roger bought a CD. We went to a pizza place and I ate the least expensive pizza. A humble Margherita. All my economizing was in vain. Roger spent money because he wanted the crowns spent.

I saw a picture of two women kissing and felt an overwhelming desire to be kissed by some man. No man has ever made love to me, and my body, which desires, is about to crack. So I calmed down and the voice, triumphant, began to irritate me, in fact the voice irritates me constantly. I can only say that since he fell for her, the voice wants me out of his way and life has become impossible. A terrible emptiness is enclosing me. Yesterday I did nothing but feel my backside, because my injected place needed scratching. I haven't had a bath in two days, and I itch.

Today I wait to go back to mother and the safety of routine. This place is now the past. I have now found the voice's weak point. I threatened to fuck Miss Beyaz and the voice is agreeable. In fact he is saying I am ungrateful, but he started it. I want revenge.

I now began to pray, and my thoughts turned again to God and my play. Roger had an idea yesterday of getting teabag paper and placing it near the door. I threw it into the bin. I'm going to be there instead. Imagination is a powerful thing..

25-05-03

Went and came back from Prague. Briefly wrote the diary but now I need to work on it and type it. Dad's chemotheraphy is painful to watch, he is a changed man but then he was always weak, prone to be a hypochondriac and then when he got ill, he changed to a passive sufferer. What is suffering? What makes a man take so much suffering while other people hardly feel pain, and why do they think it a judgment from God?

On Thursday I said something which everyone thought interesting about the state of the mental health. I said how every mental patient was now controlled except for the few who did not have drugs. This woman wrote about a mentally ill woman ringing a bell and setting off the alarm. I found it Gothic and exaggerated. Nowadays, a mentally ill patient who is stable looks after herself, and maybe others as well.

I was of course talking about a friend of mine who lives with her parents in sheltered housing accommodation, looks after her boy friend too. But last time I saw them they both looked rather thoughtful as if their lives were not what it was. She doesn't do any voluntary work except perhaps as a protest.

I sometimes think that mental illness is a bizarre tool we use not to live our lives in our limited means. Isn't that what a mentally ill person does, protesting about not living life in a manner befitting her grand passion of ideas?

Dad has coughed and he must be all right, because earlier in the evening before he went to bed, he had a bath and could not get out of it. This old age business is sad to see.

26-05-03

Today we had a party and we blew the candles, and ate cake and barbecue. The weather man predicted rain and we had rain, but we also had sunshine.

The voice and Miss Beyaz, I think, have had a quarrel, because this morning the voice did say that he loved her more than anyone else. I am so glad. Father is walking about in the corridor, going to the toilet and flushing it too. It is like a pasta junction. He said try and sleep, but I have been catching up with the typing, and it is nearly 1.30A.M. So I cleaned and over saw the barbecue. I cut the grass in the front door garden, and made everything as far as I was able, good and looked after. Yesterday, while walking the dog an idiot was screaming at Susie, then, when I went to a house, someone was entering the house, it could have been the household's kids. But I phoned the police and I was not taken seriously, they asked about the children, but nothing happened. So it was the household's kids.

What am I going to do with my life?

29-05-03

Today I read out my poetry to general good will. They called it Fatma's poems which seem to have Maurice stumped. Why is my poetry puzzling him when everything I have learnt should make it otherwise? I had got my arse and ass mixed up. The general incoherence is what is puzzling everyone. Why am I so scatty with language? Language is a tool I must learn to use. It was because when I was growing up my precision was lost. When abused I was told repeatedly to forget precision, and now it is telling on me. Do you know what it is like to be tortured in the privacy of your own home? Well I do, and then the massive breakdown. How could I not forget?

Then I went to Mike's class. There was a woman called Sue who came with Michel and she read two stories. I found one of them extremely interesting yet I can't remember the language she used, nor even if she was telling me something profound. It was about a mother daughter relationship, old age and how it affects us all. It was extremely powerful. I liked it.

I went to the library and used the computer. I did an 800 word short story. Then after finding myself and the story I had no more time left, and I had to stop. I had booked for an hour anyway. Then I came home, read in the garden and all seemed to be peaceful. Dad has had chemotherapy and was in pain. As night approached he could not stand it and we called the doctor who made up a prescription over the phone. It was near eleven when we set off with dad to get the prescription. Dad took his walking stick and we made our way as fast as we could, circumstances permitting.

Dad came a good deal behind me and I grew afraid that he might have fallen over in the street, and I can't lift him.

The precision of language? What is precision. I must concentrate on poor Dad. We luckily went on a 96 which took us to Welling where we got another bus. Dad painfully slow. Then off at the bus stop, and I asked where the pharmacy was, and some man told me. I think it was the voice but I was not sure. I rushed towards the bridge. There were drunks and police. There might have been a robbery. I raced and found the pharmacy, but lost myself in the darkness of the night as if it were a cloak round my shoulders.

I got the medicine and more slowly went looking for dad. He was not far off. Then there was this boy and girl outside MacDonald's, there they were feeling each other, not even love but pure lust. Also, there were two drunken ladies, who looked at the couple touching each other, and they giggled. I saw a banana peel and I avoided it. Then dad nearly stepped on it, so I put it in the bin.

30-05-03

I had a day with mixed blessings, with pain and suffering and humour. I got up, walked the dog, then tried to be educated and failed miserably. The lawn mower I could not work, it was impossible. The woman took one look at me and worked it, and for good measure she worked it again. I had spent the good part of an hour trying to work it, and she was there. I called out to the voice, but it would not budge, thinking it owned the Focus store. I am helping it. I need to buy certain things from that store so I best not forget.

The new lawn mower was even more difficult. There were too many things that needed to go into too many places. John, God bless him, came to our rescue John is our neighbour. He came and said things and sorted the lawn mower. I told him about dad's cancer and how dad had got robbed. He fixed everything. I rang the council, then the council rang us, three times. Ziynet rang three times. I answered them all.

I took Susie for a walk again, shorter than the last walk. Then had to go and pick up my photographs and read the paper, and the book, The Incredible Lightness Of Being, about the Czech Republic. But before that, I tried to clean the printer and then phoned various people. They found my name and are going to send me duplicates of the insurance...

Then I went to class and did some print making, met John and my friends, we socialized. Not the neighbour John, another John.

1-06-03

I went to the exhibition and met John there. It was a non starter. The voice is crowing away like mad because I made a fool of myself over John. Anyway the voice and Miss Beyaz are having this passionate affair, and so they do not want to be disturbed. She was on TV, her hair covered by a fur coat, not because she has done anything stupid, but she has dyed her hair and did not want the media to see.

She is having a wonderful start, what with a famous boy friend who adores her, and a mother who is my age to guide her, no, she is definitely in the lolly but is she happy? She speaks about her childhood and how fat she was.

I typed today and did some chores. I'm reading bits and pieces about the bible; you know I never realized before that the Bible is about Israel. So my day was filled with walking the dog, and being a supportive daughter and everything. Mum is doing the stairs, she is thinking that we are not clean enough, because yesterday I borrowed the lawn mower from 54, and so went into number 54's house, and saw how clean they were, so mum is jealous. She wants to be the Jones, but I don't think we can be, we definitely are all right, but if Maria dies, then I think Joe will retire and we'll have nothing.

2-06-03

I have started a play about my relationship with someone. My relationship with men has been fraught, and with the voice it has been less than perfect, I blended the two and I have a character which equals anything I have created before. I am hoping it gets performed.

The voice and I have had a really bad day. I swore at him and he swore he loved Miss Beyaz, swore he would love her forever more. Then I went and had my injection, there was blood on the toilet seat and blood on the plaster. I tried to read but could not, a terrible rage had gripped me, and I did not know what to do. When I went to the poetry café I was calm and collected my thoughts. I ordered a soup and began to worry that I would not have enough material to read. I sat alone and the voice grew distant, and I distrusted myself to think about the voice, or anything connected with emotion.

Today I have been looking at writers and their spouses, there is always one. I have the voice, true; it does all the hack work, remembering to show me the alleys, and ways to go to the Poetry Café. The voice reminded me to take my work, and reminded me about my glasses. I read a bit of the paper. Again I met Richard McKenna and he said that he is a schizophrenic too. Said he too has had the depo. It is always good to meet survivors, and become involved with them. I bought two books from Richard McKenna. I see it as an investment, I see it as life's blood.

Mother did not like me to buy all those books, she complained bitterly about me squandering my money. Dad said, "Never depend on other people."
They are both worried about me as their near end approaches I sense they are worried, but I am happy in what I am doing, and if only the voice were real I would leave him to be with his chosen people.

I am powerless about the voice because it is something I can't control, and as my death approaches I sense that I'll never be anything but a burden on the voice's conscience. If it had been a real man I would have gladly given everything that he asked for, but there is only emptiness there, misery is there, what can I do but feel the shadows are conquering, that I am losing.

Now it is night and there is so much silence, as if the noise had not happened, during the day a terrible loneliness grips my heart. Today the sun had been shining and I was alone, and my body ached with the heat, and I, to spite the voice, retreated into being mad, and said over and over,"The sun is cold." The voice got very angry about that, and on and on it went until I was nearly sick. The most pleasure I get nowadays is spitefulness against the voice.

4-06-03

I went with my books to the Big Issue, Pam was there, and she suggested I do an article about editors whom I have known, and I know a few.

In the morning on the bus a blinding flash of illumination gripped me as Jeannette sat next to me and started her business. She is a fat woman and her thigh touched mine and the voice said what a lovely thing it was. But then it was her voice which was doing it. The voices in our heads are telling us to do that as a recompense for doing our chores. I got tired of Jeannette and her suffering, so left the bus. Her thigh touching mine was warm but tiresome, I don't think I'll ever have a man but neither a woman.

I went to a lecture at the campus and enjoyed it. At the Big Issue the book is set on course. Then in the evening another woman's thigh nearly touched mine and I wound up reading the paper. I am bored with the voice's strategy, that he is moving to Turkey to be with his Miss Beyaz, and wants all his affairs neatly wrapped. Did not anyone tell him that life is not neat, that it is painfully messy?

I sometimes wonder if I am going mad. What if I end up killing or hitting one of these woman? I don't want them touching me, for heavens sake.

Sometimes I say I shall die soon and it won't matter, none of this will matter. Sometimes, as I go up and down the same road that I've been doing   for eleven years I say it does matter, because I matter. But no one in their right minds hears voices making them do these things, so I must be mad.

John Bird came to the writer's group today and said he was going to open a Big Issue in Japan. I thought he was in financial trouble? No, apparently he is not, but the vendors do say that the Big Issue is more difficult to sell.

I must go to bed now. The voice is grinning away to himself, so pleased with himself, and I don't know the reason. But then he is the most irritating voice I've had the misfortune to know.

5-06-03

I have to admit that today I went up and down stairs, carried stuff and signed contracts, and passed my foundation. So I am generally pleased with myself. It is father's chemotherapy day and father is sick. But I am, on the whole, finding myself and happy. I have been complimented on my looks by a mad man and was told in no uncertain terms that I was all right. To be told that one is all right, when the voice tells one in no less uncertain terms that I look a right drag and need a face lift, is a boost, even if the boost is by a mad man.

I realize now that I can't do anything about the voice, that we must co exist in my world and I can't go to his world. I even suggested that he take a flight occasionally to go and see theatre. The poor voice will be cooped up in Turkey, thinking about nothing but building and construction. What it is to be an older woman, one has to be older to be wiser, but I don't think one is. One can pretend to be happy, but there is always that unhappiness that sees life slipping and nothing making sense.

I started on my two essays and I hope to have them ready by Sunday so that my sister can read them. That is all from me.

6-06-03

All my days are dark and bitter. I seem to be spending dark thoughts and the voice does nothing but aggravate them. I took my 'Scream' painting and was nearly attacked by some children who told me, as I was crossing the road after posting my letter, to "Come here!" Luckily a bus passed and I grabbed it. They would have broken my 'Scream'. I was shaken and went without further incident to the college. At College Fey my teacher said, "You must do a dry point of this, it is fantastic, so much energy." I tried to do other things but then after two tries capitulated, and did what Fey wanted. It was a labour of love, but I did it.

Then the voice began. I nearly jumped underneath a train, but did not, because I wanted to hang up the exhibition. I have one more credit to get. The bus was a near thing as well. The voice says I am a lesbian and because of that Jim had not married me, because of that.

You know sometimes I would give everything to be quiet. This playing around with people's lives is getting to be past a joke. I saw Jim's new favourite and she seems to be happy. I was never happy with Jim.

Miss Beyaz on television said she wanted to be a girl for six more years and she had a crafty expression on her face. I know that they are trying for babies. All I can say is, not on my time. My hair is falling and as I looked at Miss Beyaz's I compared our heads, she seems to be offering more, so now before I die all I want is a moments peace. I want to be peaceful so I can gather my strength and weaknesses, and to be me.

8-06-03

Today I went to the Mary Ward Centre an hour late, but so were the others all an hour late, we sat and chatted for twenty minutes. My friends kept on asking about my scholarship. Then we went to find Marlyn, I met her on the staircase. I met John on the staircase too. He gave me his stories. I was touched that he sets such store by my publishing him. Some of his writing is powerful, and some just boring. But he is such a gentle man. I wish he could have kissed me. I think he is shy. Well so am I. I haven't ever physically kissed a man, not since Angel.

I have been thinking about my life and how Angel destroyed my life because of the party, and how James objected to my being kissed by Angel. Any other man would have knocked Angel and carried me off. But Jim only nagged for twenty one years, then found other women to satisfy him and the reason he did not marry me was, so he says, my lesbian tendencies.

It was various factors I guess, but I am still a virgin, so who knows, I might find someone else! Youth, I think, is glorious. I saw Miss Beyaz on TV, a beauty if ever there was one, but brainless. Maybe she has artistic flair. Anyway Jim's current girl friend is the woman he wants to make his wife. I give them six years of contentment and bliss, then, when she becomes thirty and he fifty odd, I think they'll become like Jim and me now. God, in six years time I'll be fifty.

I wanted to die today and I could not help the threats I made, and the many things I wanted to do became pushed aside. I can't help being jealous of his happiness but what I can help is the replacement. John and I will be one, but it is finding the courage to tell him that I am petrified, and need help to give up my virginity before the voice ends up destroying me.

Belgin and Roger came today, Roger says there is nothing the matter with the printer. So tomorrow I have to buy a new ribbon. I read the Bible and reread certain things which I had not pondered for thirty years. The trees and the months in the Revelation is great, it is not fiction. But then I understand why Israel is important and why Jews think they are important...

10-06-03

Today has been a mad rush of activity. Fiona calls me a whirling Devrish and today I have proof that that is what I am. Fiona is from the Big Issue, she is so timid and brow beaten, having suffered the normal share which is everyone's lot. I see her at the Help desk as she charitably goes about her business. She has a dread of Frances. Frances is the boss and she doesn't like me, the first thing she did was to fire me from my unimportant job. Now I do a bit of voluntary work for them. It is on the cards that I won't be doing it for much longer, I am running out of poetry to read to the writers group.

Mum's leg is hurting her. She has green on it. The nurse took a sample, which she normally does. Mum has been over doing it and soon I will have to take care of her..

The voice has been very active as I painted, he was still as I sculpted, and I got mad with a mad bubbling laughter. When I try to do my own face I can't do so. Miss Beyaz was on the news and she is the sexiest woman in Turkey, not because she is, but she believes she is, and having a rich lover does help. All the Turkish women are green with envy, and the men want her, one can see the men slurping her name.

Sex is a thing one can't eat with a spoon; one has just got to dive in. The voice tried to make me into a lesbian and I don't want to, I just want to be safe and sound next to a man. I don't understand why? My heart is giving in. I am not becoming a lesbian but my heart is aching, there is something wrong with it, it is all so stupid really, but I am in a boiling rage all the time... I am scaring all my friends.

Roger could not fix the printer. I am without a printer now for a month. Luckily I am not reading as much as before.

12-06-03

Today I've decided that I will not eat. I just won't eat, it is because of the voice. Last night I went to class and a girl asked, "Do you want to walk to Stratford." So I said okay. She walked so fast, her shoes were maniac, she must have been half a mile in front of me. She just went. Then she disappeared. I don't like that sort of friendship, did she have a whip? I just see her with a whip, whipping everyone to a pulp.

I want none of that. A man would be agreeable, maybe Gerry or John? The voice is bragging about his perfect Miss Beyaz. I wonder if there is such a perfect Miss Beyaz, or if I've made it up? I gave in two essays yesterday. I wanted to make it more perfect, (the essays). Days are passing, every time I pray I have visions of splendour, of a presence of peace. The trouble is I don't pray enough.

Today I had a vision about growing old, why we grow. Why, everybody asks, do we grow old if God loves us? Suddenly I knew if we did not grow old we would do to each other all manner of wrong, because there would not be fear. We live in fear of growing old, which is why we don't do wrong. When a child is growing it knows no fear, when the young adult goes and does sport it fears nothing, but as we age we grow. Our perceptions grow.

13-06-03

Today is Friday and I've just been painting or trying to. I have a great deal of painting to do. A terrible anxiety is besetting me. I look haggard and old. The voice is making me impotent, by the time I argue with the voice all my desires are over. I want revenge. He is going to lose his Miss Beyaz if he persists in trying to make me into a lesbian.

Tonight I might tell my mother what he's been doing. I have to, she is my rock. We did the garden today and I was happy. If I become a recluse the voice will stop. But many years of arguing with the voice and I am old. I feel old. I don't desire anyone, why because I am on medication and the voice thinks that I am a lesbian. He wants to know why? Because of the medication.

I have accepted that I'll never marry, but the voice is being like a man drunk with love for Miss Beyaz. Because of her he wants everyone to have sex. I think after the exhibition I'll end it all. My hunger strike did not go well. I had revulsion against food that was all. Then I ate more than ever.

Went to print making and saw John, and did a good print. Sat with blind Jane. Her dog likes me and expects to find food. I like dogs. Now I am on my way home. Feeling terribly tired. I am the ugliest woman on this planet. I feel it and look it. I look severe, and always tired.

15-06-03

Yesterday I learnt that James is living with the perfect Miss Beyaz. Now I am calm again and have realized that no man will have me because I am different. I am nothing. I have nothing left. Now I sit and think. If music be the food of love? No, it is not music, it is beauty that is the food of love, without beauty there is nothing but empty years of waste, waiting and cringing, one more year has passed but no one is coming, and even if they did, they are different, and you are not the innocent girl you were.

Life is terrible. I am afraid of being alone, like a shower I run on and on.

We went to the park today and had cake. We missed father, he went out, so it was father's day without father. A terrible emptiness gripped me as if I was playing a part.

I was playing the part of auntie, a student, a daughter, and I was all these things, yet I was nothing. I did belong but I have no one to share all the parts I play. My sanity dissolves like a sieve.

I become less but no one knows, no one commented. We went on a crowded bus and a man told me to move, I felt like shouting, where? Where can I move? Then someone pushed me, did I exist? Do I exist? A terrible fear that I might be going mad has gripped me! After thinking about what I have written, a fear of the world and what it can do! The voice did say it preferred me mad because I was more manageable. I don't want to be mad again, being mad everyone ignores one, and one is not even a fly. Like the family keep on looking to see if I am all right.

We were celebrating dad's being cured of cancer, but dad just disappeared. You see he is mad too. Ziynet's foundation is going well, I have almost finished my foundation. It's time I relaxed.

17-06-03

Today I did class after class. Yesterday I painted a 6 foot by six foot picture. I am very pleased with it. Today I cut myself and the blood just flowed. It was in the sculpture room. No one saw me for I had become invisible. But the week after they said something about it which gave me a jolt.

The voice is still on about his sex life, and how he wants to sort everyone out and give me a woman. He makes me feel sick I ever thought he was a man to be trusted and depended on. I think he'll get what he deserves.

Days and days go and I haven't done anything but quarrel with myself, the voice, and the dog. I am impotent. I am impotent.

Yesterday I found that his Miss Beyaz is hard, so is he, but she is harder. She'll eat him whole, and he wants that. She said that a woman should not be juggling monkeys. Yes, but that is what women do. They are always juggling monkeys, since time began. So what makes a hard woman turn womanly? Love, she is not in love with him.

19-06-03

Yesterday I went to university and was touched by a man. It was a great moment for me. The lecture was about Gaia. Importantly, I asked a great many questions. Tomorrow I am going to the university library to see about getting a book. Today Jaime took us to Tring and we were stuffed silly with food, I drew and talked with people, and had a lovely time. Jaime opened the toilet door by mistake and I was in it. We were both embarrassed. He said I should lock the toilet door. He reminded me of dad.

Then I asked him when we could book the Diorama gallery. He said any time, and then he said we'll discuss it next week.

I had an interesting conversation with Veronica, it was bizarre, all about her illness and George Bush. I wonder if George Bush is her voice? Well James is mine. I just wonder, that is all.

Later I had an interesting discussion with a man. He said he did not need a house.
"I am saving money, I am earning a living, I don't need anything. I have been painting for six months and I don't need tuition. I also don't need a mortgage. I signed three homes to my former wife and I don't need a thing!"

I am surrounded by people whose values are so different. I felt apologetic because I did not believe a word of it. But this man was looking 25 and he was 45. Then the voice looked eagerly at all the women, sizing them up for me. A terrible boredom beset me, like I did not like him, as if I would strangle him if I could. I am writing this on my way back from Tring and on the whole it was a good trip, as if I have become a human being after all.

30-07-03

On the holiday journey we had a nasty jolt. Travelling became a nightmare of trying to keep calm while dad wet himself in front of everyone. He and a diabetic woman kept the toilet occupied. One would go and then the other. But dad was more frequent. On the journey to Kyrenia, he was jolted, his ego sank to a low, and he became so cross he was impossible. He was so angry with us for dragging him to Cyprus, for giddying about and flaunting ourselves like whores. He had a pill to calm himself.

Dad complained about lack of urine when he wanted to go, mercifully we arrived and he went to bed, but he could not sleep. He would stop the coach and go, he stopped the coach so frequently that the coach driver was angry. But the man, who was Oktay, was sympathetic. Dad was so cross. I was feeling guilty, it was no one's business. I commented that dad looked as white as a sheet. Dad said he was no longer a beauty.

Now, today, he sleeps, after wetting two swimming trunks and yesterday's trousers. I took a taxi and went for food. I had to make an effort for a good holiday.
Parents are asleep and my cousin is coming to see him.

I said to Yucel, my cousin, that dad was very ill, could he come over. Now he has become better, regaining his sense of humour. Mum, poor thing, had to bath dad all by herself. She could not shower so I put a chair and took her leg off. Her artificial leg must not get wet, otherwise she would not be able to walk. This holiday is fast becoming a Kafka-like nightmare.

Dad woke up to just escape wetting the bed, but his feeble stumbling was not enough and again he was wet. He got entangled in the bed clothes. A terrible struggle ensued. I rescued dad. It was too late. We had an argument about penicillin. He needs some antibiotics but he won't take any.

Finishing that argument he went to bed and I am writing this. I think I'll go for a walk.

31-07-03

This is the final day of the month. A peaceful kind of acceptance has invaded me. People are eating their sandwiches, these are feta cheese and toast. The sea is opposite us. A thousand messages, I accept that I am me, not a lesbian, and that I will never marry because the voice won't let me.

I won't be sad. As the sun shines, a terrible acceptance that life does not go on, and I wish the voice might die in a car crash. That I too might die but I love life.

Mum is in pain, her shoulder hurts. Dad's legs are swollen and I feared the worse. Yucel, my cousin came with his family. The toilet is stinky, because dad has started to wet the floor, and he has a smell which is disgusting. I also wet myself because I have my period.

Dad is better. My cousin yesterday did not write the address down, so was wandering the road to find us. When he came he was sleepy. Cousin's wife was okay, their children grown up. How fast children grow!

I told the cleaner to clean the toilet. Now I feel almost clean but I am a mess. Today I went to Kyrenia and got lost. But I would not get a taxi. I paid the outward journey, 8000,000. I bought dad slippers. He is more comfortable. He constantly wets himself. He needs to be reminded of the room number.

When I was in Kyrenia he went to the wrong room, the woman began to shout. I'm going away for a day, I just wonder who will look after them. I'm going to the Greek side, and to a Turkish wedding.

1-08-03

I had to call the doctor. The doctor turned out to have been a neighbor of Dad's. Dad said he had a pretty white wife. The doctor was old. His bedside manner was excellent. This morning I went and got his pills. I thought all the chemists would be shut, because it is a celebration of the Turkish Liberation Day. So I thought I would be stranded. The hotel person said take the Dolmush and go to Kyrenia, which I did, and found a chemist very quickly. I waited while two women discussed their prescriptions. Then one of the

woman said she could not walk without her
Ibupform.

Got Dad's medicine, paid 19,000,000. I was
so glad, and told the chemist that I thought
everything would be closed. The chemist said he
could not afford to be closed. Went on the
Dolmush after asking the chemist where I should
board. The journey was pleasant, with music, and
the people all squeezed into a small van, about
ten people. The hotel I found very quickly.
Karaoglan, which is the one after the supermarket.

I was pleased with myself, after a short
walk I was at the hotel. Breakfast was not long. No
second cup of tea. Dad got better. Mum and Dad
are virtual prisoners. I went again to the shops,
bought more food. Kebab for dad, and yet he had
oily food. His diabetes is out of control. I slept and
became hotter than ever. At night I asked about
going to the Greek side, no, was the answer, not
with a British passport. I don't believe them, I'm
going tomorrow.

Dad's waiting for his food and I think
someone who works in the hotel fancies me. I am
too bruised.

3-08-03

We are in the hotel room, dad keeps
spitting into the sink. The hotel was alive
yesterday, full to the brim with rich people. The

hotel was like a young girl all dolled up. The music and the singing and people chattering went on until late. Mum said the waiters ate at four a.m. We also went, but they made it obvious that serious money must be spent, we left as soon as we ate the kebabs, which were very small portions. Dad always goes to the loo.

The hotel owners' son screwed a young woman. I've grown used to it. Every man that I ever met screwed other women in front of me. I went shopping today, bought antibiotics for mum. I bought a powder for dad and some painkillers, total, thirty one million lira. Then I bought tweezers.

The day passed hot and humid, it was so hot that I could not move, went and slept. Mum did not want to go to dinner so I took dad. Dad went upstairs to mum to get his injection and got lost, he was lost for half an hour. I did not realize until he was well away from the hotel. Mum came down and I was near the sea where the shack restaurant was, flirting and thinking. The hotel keeper found him. Dad was very thirsty. He drank four glasses of water.

4-08-03

In the middle of our holiday I've found nothing but never ending me. The hotel is surrounded by rich dames. Oktay is spoilt for choice. I think he is in bed with the blonde with the dog. Now a dark haired woman is waiting for him.

There is no room for me so I'll just laugh with no one in particular. I'll be okay. I know men so well, especially if they have money. I met a nice guard who showed me round and bought me lemonade. He was so enthusiastic about the museum, so polite, and he showed me the museum in a way that appealed to me.

Dad lost his way again. I found him. We asked the waiters' wages and he said if he got married his wages would not be enough. So in other words he is looking for a rich wife, namely me. If only he knew, I am not rich.

5-08-03

Today the heat entered me in a dismal fashion. I had seven cokes. I tried to write, I tried. I could not concentrate because my limbs felt dead and I had a painful headache. I could not get rid of the headache. I had a premonition of not being able to write forever. I wrote two poems which passed the time.

Dad had said on the plane that Cyprus, his homeland, had smelt of home, now he can't wait to go back to England. I know why I feel so out of sorts. I think I am involved with a man.

Every Turk I ever met complains about the Greeks. That the Greeks don't spend money, that they buy drinks and have packed lunch. Now we talk about my dead uncle, how he said that dead man's property is for the taking. I wonder if my cousin feels the same? He came with his family looking concerned for dad. He sat with his big head and balding body as if he were about to conquer the world. He looked older and tired. He looked rough, a work man, not a gentleman.

Miss Beyaz is very famous. But I shan't think of it, that is a stupid private agony, a disease. All that I want now is to live. I must live.

6-08-03

Phoned my sister, we chatted about the cats, she said everything was all right in England. I went to pay for the phone in the reception area, I saw Oktay as he looked through the phone bill. I paid. He appears to be nice. His mother is bored. I want to be nice to her. How can I love him? I don't know him. We have five days of our holiday left.

I must not lose control or my dignity. But I feel so happy to be with a man who thinks I am pretty, and does not compare me to a sex goddess. The voice has stopped tormenting me. Maybe this holiday has stopped the voice for good.

7-08-03

I had a day filled with life, a day full of joy and sadness. First, we ordered a cab. The cab came late. Just as the cab came who should come but Durmush my cousin? He came larger than life. I kissed him on the cheeks. Oktay's brother, the cab driver, reasoned as we sat in the cab. Oktay is a jealous man. I explained about Durmush being like a brother to me. He is a double cousin and I've known him since time began. Hate his wife though, and this looked bad.

We arrived at aunt Fetine's house. Oktay's brother stayed and waited for us. Aunt tried to make us stay for the night. Dad wanted to get back to the hotel, and I to Oktay. Dad only stopped the car once. I took everyone's photo, and we had to say goodbye.

Dad got granddad's walking stick, it looks strong. He can't walk without his walking stick. Aunt, a widow has her husband's cap and walking stick on the wall. The room is large and the roof leaks, but aunt sleeps in the other house, and she uses this house to cook and look after her grandson. She is so sad about uncle's passing, but she is waiting to join him and she is being useful at the same time.

We all went to the toilet, it is a large room with no door, but it is within the bedroom, so people in the living room can't hear, or maybe they can but they don't see one. Our brief visit was over. Aunt reluctantly said good bye, and I was relieved because I wanted to be with Oktay.

I chatted about this and that all the way through the journey, but I wish I had never spoke to the driver, for he followed me afterwards and Oktay was jealous.

Dad has constipation and so do I. Then I met the mum of Oktay and his sister in law, his brother's kid. Not the taxi driver, but his older brother. They asked about me and I was the centre of attention. I might have to emigrate to Cyprus. I have to do away with the voice.

8-08-03

Oktay sent a message that he wants to talk to me before commitments, and he wants to know me. I had not realized that we had not talked. I went to the sea, seething, throwing weeds in the air. I read Victor Hugo. Oktay played a game. I conceded. He was absolutely right. We talked at the bar for two minutes, and he asked me questions he knew the answers to. There was the gay waiter as well. Oktay beat him. I bet the waiter allowed that. He is no fool, he tried to read my diary. The diary is the only reality I have. Oktay says he won't allow me to be lost, but he is so laid back that I will be lost.

12-08-03

From the warmth and hope of thinking one is loved, and wondering if one should sell up and go to him, and be with him forever and forever, one's life is stretched in effortlessness and warmth. No, it did not happen like that. He was in the bar eating his food and when he saw me he did a funny shake of the head, like a horse, or a young man who is always busy and needs to be quiet with himself. I asked him if he cared and he said he was off on a holiday with his wife.

They are going to Antalya for a week. So now I am on a plane going back to what I do best: WORK. Next month I start university. I am torn between going back there to see him again, and repulsion at myself. I just wonder if it is all my imagination, did he ever love me?

We had talked. I talked to his family. I never saw his wife. I just wonder if he made her up. He does not love me. I want so much to have him, his delicious body, his sharp brain, the way he aggressively moves, but he said he was running a business and that was why he was kind to me, today his dad could not wait to see the back of us. I just loved him so.

23-08-03

Painted mum, painted scenery, wrote poems. Everything I do I think of him, Oktay. I think he is watching me but he is in Cyprus, no, how could he? I think as I read the paper, should I go to him? Remember he is married. I feel less already. I have forgotten his face. Only his dear body and his last words I remember. He said he was running a business and being nice was his business.

I walked the dog and lazed round. My grant money allocation came. Everything will start. I'll give poetry lessons. My confidence in my ability has gone. Why do I always go for the wrong guy?

24-08-03

The dog is barking. Dad is in bed wearing old pyjamas. I have decided what to do with me. I want a doctorate. I want to write, I must write. An acceptance of me has paralysed me. I accept that I am a woman whom no one wants. I am too ugly, also that I am old. I am set in my ways. I bow in acceptance.

The voice has raised its head in glee but, having fallen in love I know that I don't fancy women. I never will. Miss Beyaz was on television, in a filthy temper. The voice desires her so much like he never desired me. I accept that my shadowy world is a habit that will always be a habit, but it can't hurt me like it used to do. Miss Beyaz is a child playing with her toys.

I've had a break, was aroused, if only Oktay were older and unmarried, but one can't have a man married to someone else. In Cyprus I read poems by Victor Hugo in Turkish, in London I am reading again. I want to be a doctor of art. Why? To give myself confidence, to bolster me. To get this flagging ego moving in the right direction. I hope that the voice is not standing in my way as he had previously. I have been an arrogant miss, and the voice had said if you love me you'll not go to university, and he pulled my world out of its socket.

He would not allow me to study! Why? Because only when I study, do I become alive. Now Miss Beyaz and he can go to hell because in my world there is no room for flops. Miss Beyaz shows off a terrible tiredness of the rat race, of her constant bickering with other stars, and her desire to be at the top at any price. I wonder what do men want?

Do they want bad temper and bile or do they want order, serenity, and not a dolly bird?
Life is a sadness when one realizes that one cannot accept everything lying down. Loudness and as one bangs into the limelight, that is not everything. One must have quiet. I can now think. I must celebrate my life for no one else will. I am a writer, an artist. I am a woman, an artist with a book contract. I am also alone.

I have calculated 7 years later I will be 52. I will be all right. I'll have books, exhibitions, things will happen, nice things. Maybe it was never love what I felt. Maybe it was never anything but fancy, if only it were real love I would have left me behind and gone to him, I would have helped him. I wanted him so.

Oktay refreshed me, showed me that I was not bad to look at, and showed me what a man can achieve in a short time. Then he ran away, said he was married! Married! What I've lost I don't know, but he helped me gain my womanhood. He was my Valentine and everything. He was also everybody's, I wonder, was he a whore. Did he sleep with all the guests?

He did not sleep with me. I offered, but he did not. I offered twice, he refused both times. I thought he was mine, that it would be all right, nothing has gone right. I was certain he followed me to England, for weeks I was in a holiday mood. But no, he was not. I have to accept the fact that I was not even amusing.

25-08-03

I got up feeling my day was too short, that I could not possibly fit it all in! Walked the dog, read the paper, and I am reading a book "A Room with a View". We invited the sisters on a picnic. I wore my jacket, it was warm. Ziynet objected to the jacket so I took it off. Then everyone started to go to the toilet and I went with them. Dad went first, he chose the wrong way so I pointed the right way, but just in case he got lost I went with him. Little Ted was playing football with Belgin, he was sweating. Leyla and David were playing hide and seek. I have not known such peace in years.

I sat and ate Roger's pasta, the spinach was not washed properly, Belgin ate and ate. Yesterday they both had mud right to their knees and rescued themselves. Those two are adventurous. One or the other will do something in the way of adventure. I said nothing and we sat until daylight was less intense, we sat until I was totally at peace.

Dad got restive, then he said, "You are such a liar!" And he left. I wondered if he would lose his way, the day's peace was shattered, broken into fragments. Ziynet, assuming a busy air, said, "I have to go to my car because the traffic warden is probably there, waiting for me to leave the car longer."

David, my five year old nephew had wandered off, but we were too busy discussing how many acres of land we had. The decision is I go next year, sort everything, and do something about it. The deeds are what we want, and we have only two acres for the deeds. David, the little chap came and without a word, sulked.

It was time to leave, so we took everything and separated after Roger and Belgin debated whether to get a zone four bus or not. Belgin did not have a ticket for zone four, only for zone 3. In the end they decided to walk it.

Mother and I got on 53 bus. Mother sat where the prams are, and I sat at the back, my plates juggling as I made myself comfortable. Some more people got on and I was less comfortable. They seemed unsure of their destination. The man kept on jumping up and sitting on different seats.

We arrived at Woolwich, the plates juggling and cluttering, we went home. I did not want dinner; dad had been to a café to feed his diabetes. From the garden I picked apples. Then mum fell, food all over her hair, broken plates, and dad waiting for his dinner. I had been doing the syringes and I rushed over. Mum edged near the sofa and I lifted her up.

"I don't know what made me fall!" she said, "It must have been something in my way." The dog ate the food, I shooed it away. Dad demanded his food. Mum's confidence is at its lowest. She was not badly hurt. We put cream on the leg. Then we cleaned everything up. Gave dad his food. We watched T.V. Afterwards Ziynet rang.

"My mother-in-law's lung has collapsed and the thing they put in has made her body swell. From looking thin she looks terrible." And she began to cry.
"I'm leaving the kids with you. We don't know whether she will live or die."

So the kids are coming to us. I'm taking them shopping and to MacDonald's, that is tomorrow.

Maureen is better. Her swelling is going down. Her sons and daughters and grand children are with her. I put salty water and mum bathed her leg, she too is better.

27-08-03

I lost my temper with my little nephew David. I hit him on the head three times. He hurt Leyla's eye. Ziynet says Leyla lies, and my nephew is not speaking to me like he used to. That night, Leyla came and slept in my bed while I slept on the floor, she could not stop laughing. She said she was not going to allow me to sleep until she had her revenge. At ten I slept. In the morning I had a bath, a time for me. I was determined on not losing my control again. Ziynet came while I was still in the bath. She took the children pretty quick.

I was over the moon to see them go. Kids, who wants to have three kids screaming at them? But I wish I had not hit my little nephew. I taught Leyla about putting on cream and things, David was thoughtful.

Today I taught poetry or creative writing. I gave some basic tips on writing, and two poetry outlets for Gail, who is a poet. Then I lost my temper with mum. My nerves so jumbled, my world upside down. I need to feel other than imposed upon. I am tired. Hopefully, tomorrow I can have the hall for the exhibition.

I miss Oktay so much, as if I am going to be a dried stick forever more because he rejected me, or played games with my feelings. I feel as if I can't give anymore.

29-08-03

Yesterday I went to the art group, nothing, not even a sausage, empty, dull, they've all gone on holiday. Today I phoned Jennifer, she did not reply. I figured I did a lot of housework, like the laundry, and made lunch, washed up, emptied the bins, until the mindless activity made me go to the phone. Somebody phoned about poetry, I tried to answer but the line went dead.

This mindless toil, housework wives do all the time. I will go mad if I have to sit at home and think, I want ceaseless intellectual activity. I want to read. I am still reading A Room with a View by Forster. I am enjoying it. I am on page 122. But what is the point of me reading? What is the point of life, when I'll not amount to anything. I am a failure in life, a terrible fate of being buried alive awaits me. I am a secret. I am a woman whom no one wants enough to over ride their objections! So what is the point of me coming alive over holidays, only to sleep again the rest of the year?

Daily I wrestle with myself, daily I win my objections. I am not rich, I can't think ahead. I can't leave everything and go after a married man. Besides, the weather there is far too hot.

This diary is my friend, I tell it everything, yet if a reader saw me they would not recognise me, for I am still alive and secret. I have not put everything of me into this diary. I challenge anyone to know me.

30-08-03

Today is like massive impressions, films, I've seen Angela's Ashes. I enjoyed the film. We went out; mother's first outing since she fell. She walks so slowly now. We stole the money from dad. He did not even notice it. In a week my benefit will be cut. You know I don't care.

Back to today's impressions, it has been a relaxed day. I did a bit of housework, cleaned the dust off the kitchen plant, put curtains up, made coffee. I am bored, or tired of having nothing to do.

I have lazed all my life. My mind has been inactive, cooking and poetry does not fill all the time one has. It's time I learnt to do better pictures. What with the TV, I had no chance to look at Room with a View. On holiday I wrote poetry, but today I've had an idea for a short story, and I am not doing it. Why should I write and be despised? Why? But I've joined a short story writing workshop so I will write for that.

1-09-03

I missed a day. Mr Perfect and Miss Beyaz have separated. Now the voice wants me to be perfect. I was looking at a video, and enjoying the feel good factor when the voice begun to make remarks about being jealous. How much longer will I be sane with that bastard in my head? How many more years?

I will never be perfect, I am not youthful, I am not beautiful, I was never beautiful. But the voice is jealous and it escalates, it goes like it has arrived at a dirty party it was not invited to, and it has been hurt. All those years and still I suffer, and am likely to go on suffering because I don't give a damn anymore.

The voice is crap, he is interested in a dancer, he wants a perfect looking woman. But does perfection exist? No, perfection in living people does not exist. No one is perfect. I want to potter about, I'll not love again, it is too late for me, but maybe the voice maybe can be perfect. The necrophilia thing.

Maybe I'll never be an interesting woman. I am 44 and still a virgin! Why? Why? Why me? I should be the one who is angry, I am the bloody wronged individual. Why me? What is there in me that brings out the worse in men?

The voice had this glorious affair and now just because the affair has ended he thinks he can order me about! Well he can think again..

I am no longer the timid girl that I had been at 24. He refused to marry me because I said women on television looked beautiful. I must admit that I was pretty screwed up, but when I told the doctor he said most women thought that way about other women, straight women. I don't see the attitude that he has, why this clinical attitude? He reminds me of Cecil in A Room with a View. He has no light; I need to be with someone who has light. He will destroy me. Already I am feeling suicidal. What is it with rich people, why are they so screwed up? He has a thing about gold diggers, at least he gets perfection every time. This time he suffered, and he was on his best behaviour, may it last a life time for him.

3-09-03

The year is nearly over, my life is getting exciting, things are snowballing. I am in the happy position of having an offer of an exhibition space. I have to ring Robert at the end of the week. I must get painting. I had gone off to the Big Issue, sorted the proofs, and then I went to Tate, because every art student must go to the Tate or the National. Then I went to an opening night of John Cahill.

John; grown dignified by his achievement. I spoke to Robert who asked if I painted, I said yes I did. Suddenly he flashed a card, call me about an exhibition he said.

I could not stop talking all night, I spoke and talked, I tried to be witty but I was not. The voice grew irritated, I expanded. I spoke to complete strangers about the course I am going to do, about my achievements. Poor things, they listened. Then I used the loo, spoke to two women, it felt oddly like work.

Today I remember, tomorrow I'll remember. Every day flashes of my past come, and I admit I do now have a past. Brief glimpses of what I was and the competent Miss I am now, but one false move and I end alone, depressed, suicidal.

Tomorrow I am going to Jaime's to book everything. I need help with choosing the pictures.

4-09-03

I carried three paintings, two of them large. Jaime liked them. Then I made green paintings, but Jaime said not to paint green always because it looks like wall paper. I spoke to Roberts' secretary, and Jaime gave social care my number. Poor people must wait at the whims of rich people.

At the National gallery Collin gave an interesting lecture. Then I asked the value of a painting, Collin said if no one wants to buy a painting then it's valueless, I persisted, and he said thirty pounds for the wood.

I wonder was he lying about the medieval painting? Then he showed us perspective, and I find perspective very difficult to get my head round.

After the lecture I was on tenterhooks about booking the exhibition. So without coke I and Jaime went to the Crypt. Lucien the man who organises and books events was not there, so Jaime said he would phone me at the weekend, maybe Saturday. I had to be content with that.

I went to get my free drink and Jaime went I don't know where. At the National café I started talking politics, we discussed Tony Blair and Campbell, was the Iraq war justified? I said it was not and that Tony Blair had the killer instinct. I also said I was voting Kennedy, The Liberals. I like the commonsensical way he talks, also I can't stand the Tories because they believe in God, and there was something about them praying every moment of each day to win the general election. I think they've lost it.

Uncle said I should stay at home and look after mum and dad. Why didn't uncle do that to with his parents? He hopped it pretty quick.

6-09-03

I got up and went to the loo. Mum has started to moan about dad. A moan that goes on and on. Dad has not slept under the covers, he mumbled that he was cold. Yesterday I took dad to be scanned for cancer and he lost his temper. He started to justify himself, and as we sat next to each other he edged nearer and nearer until I could have screamed. Then I insisted mum and dad and I go to the Chinese place to eat.

We all ate up, then mum told dad that he was old. He began to moan that he can't get away with anything! Poor mum, to be married to a mad man. He is like a child and he has no memory, and the harm he does. I wish he was dead.

Children stay married to their parents by ties stronger than any other ties. I am a child of that marriage and it's time I grew up.

7-09-03

I went to bed at 2.30 A.M and woke at 7 A.M. I have not read, my head feels like a sieve. I have a terrible fear that I am losing my life. I went to the pharmacy and got father penicillin.

Took Susie for a walk, we were both subdued. I am losing my life again. Like when I was a teenager and somebody copied my story, then the school blamed it on me. I am losing it. Those were my thoughts as I walked the dog. A depression akin to despair dampened me.

Then I saw the tree as it is, against the charred background fighting to reinstate itself, and a bliss over came me. A bliss I experience every time I look at nature when walking the dog. Then two dogs began to bully Susie so I called her over and we sat down, and I looked at the charred beauty, that is the best in London, and I thought how nature repairs itself, even as I have. The dogs came again so I quickly scampered.

We went home and I cooked sausages, the children came and ate it. Mother did us proud too. Father could not walk which dampened our spirit. Then he wet himself in front of everyone. He could not walk fast enough to the loo.

Ziynet and Mum tried to get him upstairs. A terrible struggle ensued. Finally he made it upstairs, he was burning. Ziynet and Ted took Susie for a walk, Susie likes them. Belgin is not packed and she is going on holiday in two days time.

After they left I phoned the doctor, then I caved in and called an ambulance, I am writing this in a small cubicle in casualty. But I am disturbed in every way; people come and gape at father as he lies asleep. He has wet himself and I feel painfully shy. I have seen father nude. He is not himself.

8-09-03

Yesterday I went to bed at 1.30 A.M. There were drug addicts trying to use the phone, trying to stop the taxi. It was night, beware of the night. Today was relatively uneventful. Father is to have a bed. He is still waiting in a ward in casualty.

Ziynet blamed me for not finding out about the scan, but I want to forget about the scan, it was the scan which caused father to go to bed without covering up.

Mother too went to hospital, but now I realise that father is not essential to my comfort or happiness. But of course I should not say so, otherwise if he dies I'll feel guilty.

I remember the ambulance man's words; he had lost his father when his father was 38. I've had my father for a long time, if he goes he goes and it won't be a tragedy, but an acceptance of life, life is like that.

9-09-03

I had an interview and gave 17 paintings and prints. Then I went to hospital with my folder after phoning mum. She was not there, and I went to hospital worrying that she might fall or something. Mum's birthday today.

I went to casualty to see dad's place filled with an old woman with bruises. I asked the nurse where he was and the nurse said ward 20. I walked with my folder and found dad. He was lying in a state, "How are you dad?"

"Fine, no, I'm ill."

I waited, and then went to casualty to get mum. She was not there, dad was not bothered, I was worried in case she fell. After ten minutes it was one o'clock, I went to lunch. There was a huge queue so I ate as fast as I could, there was hardly any cheese and I had paid £2.20p.

I lingered, and when I went back, there was mum in a dither trying to remember phone numbers and things with the nurse.

"Physiotherapy, and does he have a rail on the bath etc etc?"

"Yes he does!"

"He needs a shower, also a nurse. I am going to university!"

Throughout the day I kept on saying that. The more I said it the closer it became.

My leg was aching me. Then a nurse appeared out of the blue with a white jacket, "There is nothing wrong with your father!"

"What!"

"He can move when he wants to, but he'll probably get worse."

"So if nothing is wrong with him, how will he get worse?"

"Old age, the brain!"
"He's not senile?"
And he walked off.

We were flabbergasting red. I did not know what to say, a doctor from another department came.
"We don't know if the cancer has spread to his stomach!"
He left. We too left, dad with his pain, he keeps on saying he has pain. We went to a café and Mum drank coke, I had tea. We were shocked. If dad is dying how come we aren't getting help?

Then the phone at home started. Ziynet phoned, I phoned back and we agreed to visit dad tomorrow! Then uncle phoned to wish mum a happy birthday, he won't talk to me. He thinks I should stay indoors and look after mum and dad. I think I should go to university.

I had a phone call from the university telling me I should start on Monday. I have never been more disorganised. I am no way finished with my paintings. I look forward to the course.

10-09-03

Today I went to the Big Issue and said good bye. I felt terribly sad and came out with a lump in my throat and unwell. I spoke to Theo about the writing group, how it needed new blood, that for a long time no new people came. Then I thought I had something printed, and went and waited for my money from Theo. No, it was not so, and a embarrassment such as I had not had ever since the last time I felt embarrassed, which was a long time ago. I left the Big Issue with no regrets.

I went home and mum reported that dad was better. I went to a very unhelpful doctor and returned home again disillusioned. That evening I ate a lot of soup. Read the paper and watched TV. Not a lot of fun, but my life, such as it is.

What life? It is just a series of events with a camera, or this diary keeping it intact. I have been trying to organise my time, what is time? It could be nothing but coming and going and seasons passing, and a terror grips me, without that ring, the wedding ring, a woman is nothing. I want to smash the mirror and remain in my thoughts as pretty as a twenty year old. I want to wear sex! I want life.

11-09-03

It's been two years today since America was attacked. What about all the other countries? But Big America is a special case with its people, dear. I heard on radio 4 about this pilot who doubled as a farmer. This man was special and I guess he will be missed, because he had done something with his life, unlike me.

America, don't expect my sympathy because you are global, you are big, you have the capacity to destroy every country, and I think you will one day. You'll say you don't need other countries and you'll conquer them. Such as Afghanistan, or, like Iraq, those countries which you made into America, without the inclination, or the energy to change properly. You are global and that power will destroy you and the world.

I don't believe in war, not any more, even hitting the cat has lost its appeal.

Today I went to the Art Group and heard Jennifer and Jaime at loggerheads, he told her not to go to the Art Group, actually banned her. I felt sorry for her, she had put so much effort into it all, it had been her life, and now banned. Luckily she is quite rich and so has other resources.

When good people quarrel they are more aggressive then anything. I waited for Jaime for one and a half hours in the Crypt café. Then I went to find him and heard he was at a meeting. We met Petro, and in a months time I'll know when my exhibition is. Petro had been on holiday, hence the delay.

I haven't seen Sylvia and I am worried. Sylvia is going to be the other half of the exhibition. Jaime's purse was lost. I don't know what will happen, it definitely was not Jaime's day.

I did not visit dad today or yesterday because I had to walk the dog, and dad drains me. I did two pastel drawings and one of them is lovely.

13-09-03

I tried today to do things, to get things done, but time flew and I still have not properly read the paper. I took photographs for Richard, one with the Holding, and hopefully he like them. I took 26 photographs, some good ones. One set was horrible. I pasted a drawing onto an A4 sketch book, and I phoned Marlene about collecting my stuff. I have to read, I still have not returned my library books. No, today I have been busy doing nothing.

Johnny Cash has died, and like the paper said, a great voice has been taken from us. All those celebrities dying, and the non celebrity with money buying a bit of the action. Life is hilarious, I can't remember why I wanted to be a celebrity. I will write it down. I was such a failure, I guess that I wanted success, and I think all mankind wants is to succeed. Look at father, look at mum, she was modest in her dreams and she got what she wanted.

I've got half of what I wanted. Half my dreams are a reality. I've got my career but where is love? I wish I could love someone, I wish for that more than I can say.

14-09-03

We went and visited dad. I wheeled him to the restaurant, and on top of his lunch he had a sandwich. He was heavy but I wheeled him anyway. Then, like yesterday, I wheeled mum. But today I was less ill.

I read about Hemingway in the paper, then I saw Rolf Harris and his painting programme, I liked it, but as Rolf got into painting people I fell asleep. At eight there was a programme on the soul. This fascinates me, so on and off I watched it, mum did not understand, but I have read things like this in philosophy, so I understood, but not totally. I think when scientists understand what consciousness is, there won't be a mystery about the soul.

At nine I fell into deep sleep and of course I dreamt of Oktay. Between the time I flew to England and now there is nothing but loss. I watched a scandal on Turkish TV. A Turkish star was filmed having sex with a very ugly man. I think she was a victim of blackmail. I moaned when they asked the man who had filmed them? He just shrugged, it is so easy to destroy lives.
He said that he had helped the star, if he was such a helpful man why keep the film? Why not destroy it?

15-09-03

First day at university today. Chaos, chaotic, disorganised, did not know what to do, went and had a tuna sandwich, so wasn't there when the tutor called my name. He said he marked me in. He gave us a few gallery names to visit and then dismissed us. I went to the Saatchi gallery, if only my shoes did not pinch. Saw Paula Reno, admire her work, there must be 5 pieces of hers. The Maids have a homicidal tone; even the father has that undertone. Her sinister Bride with the small gaunt tailor woman…I tried to copy and realised how inadequate I am.

Went home, had tea (mint) and relaxed. Father phoned, said he wanted to get out of the hospital. I said I would be there. Went, and saw him trying to phone me. Calmed him down but he wanted to come home.

The nurse gave the district nurse a letter. He, (The nurse) said, that she could be there by Wednesday. I do hope so, otherwise mum will lose her leg from over work. Sister will contact the social services tomorrow. I pay my fee on Wednesday. I think the first week is very difficult because one does not know what is going to happen, and one has experience, but not at university level. Any way dad is at home.

I think about the voice and the voice's love life and what the voice says, and how the voice lives, and it leaves me cold as if it is akin to an alien. The part of me that is frozen. I am frozen. I went and took my photo and I am frozen. My emotions are far away.

I write so stupid, I am not educated and I desperately want to be educated to have a place in life. But I am filled with hatred for something that is not there. Maybe was there but no longer so.

I am no longer a fool. I can think but how do I think? I think of Oktay, he is there in my heart but realise he never loved me. He should have asked me to stay and I would have. I would have given up my artistic career to be with him. But he did not love me, he never asked me to stay and be with him in Cyprus. I often wonder had he lied when he said he had a wife? But how could he lie like that? Anyway my heart is there beating away as dad urinates. I watch the world happy or sad. I went to MacDonald's and saw a couple with two children. The husband made the child scream.

I regret not having children but I had been too ill. That woman at the MacDonald's was sure unhappy looking. Ward 20, the ward dad was in, was filled to the brim with people trying to get out, and these young people unhappy about something, and they want to get out. Where do they want to go? What do they want, do they know? Dad discharged himself from the hospital, but as soon as he got home he wanted to be in again. He has this idiotic grin on his face. Dad has dementia.

16-09-03

Dad has settled in the house and his smell is there like a stinky toilet. I went to the UEL. The university is huge and I kept on losing my way, I went up and down the stairs like a lunatic.

Dad is senile and we don't know what to do with him. He does not remember his appointments or anything like facts, and mum is his slave, she gets his dinner, cleans and she nanny's him. He fills the house with his urine and when he goes out to come back, he does not use his keys, but bangs on the door in an insistent manner which annoys mum. We don't know what to do. The district nurse does not either.

"He does not obey!" And mum poor mum is left at 64 to take care of a husband she pities.
I have my cheque so I can stay on at the UEL. It would not have been feasible without that as my money is running out.

I spent £80 this week. I don't know where the money has gone to. I must go and find my scholarship form, so I can cash yet another cheque next month. Life is becoming easier and I am always complaining because I mean to do this, I mean to fare well.

17-09-03

Had a row with mum, she said as she was 64 she could not exercise. I replied she was too fat, not fit. I told her the story of a man who was an overweight waiter, and I said why does she not swim?

"What, with one leg?" she has effectively shut herself in her prison.

I am reading the life story of Henry Moore. I have left everything so late, Henry Moore was 21 when he had begun his degree, plus he had been teaching. I am old! Old! I need my computer so I can work from home.

I enrolled today, then John and I went to an exhibition of someone called Allah, I forget the first name, but Feyzla, something like that. At first I was disorientated. Then I became acclimatised, I did not understand the space and the disorientation until I tried to explain to mum. Then it hit me it, was all about my reaction to it, and our response to it all, the architect and I guess, the maker, I thought I did not like it, but there is a difference between feeling nothing and feeling something.

I banked the cheque. I paid the council tax with mum's invalidity money and ordered some prescription for mum. She was up in arms saying she could not collect it from a strange chemist. She wanted to go to her own chemist. Don't old people make one ill?

She and I had another quarrel, so I told her to eat shit.

I took Susie to the park and she was all right until I began to feed her. Then she began to growl at some dog, luckily she was on a lead and so could not do anything about it.

Tired, I went home. Read Henry Moore's biography, then mum said why not make some tea, which I did, then 11.30 p.m. dad must have coffee so I told him to make it himself, which he did, grumbling that I was not a human being. So I said neither was he!

Going to university has made me outspoken. I am no longer a mouse.

18-09-03

I want to make it up with David. I miss the kids. Belgin had a dangerous holiday, for ten days she has been in Sardinia. The roof of her tent got blown and they got wet. Belgin and Roger had camped near the sea. Belgin in turn had constipation for five days. Before she went I had told her it may rain, but it seems it has poured on them.

I went to two exhibitions today, Martin Westwood, and the Whitechapel gallery, yesterday I had read a bad review on the Whitechapel one. I thought the Westwood was clear, but the Whitechapel's bad review was well deserved.

I went with the group after listening to some jokes from the fun and games at the campus. Sue, after we went to Westwood, said she would come with me. She lost her way, and my feet painful, I could just about crawl. Blisters, and it was cold, and I had on a summer dress. After drawing Westwood's stencils, I did not have the stomach for penis' erections and a man sucking a cock. Sue and I discussed family commitments and being a woman.

Family commitments erodes the artist. I agreed, she has grown up children, her daughter is 32 and she is a grandmother. Her face is huge and she is a sweetie. She also has a handicapped daughter whom she says she loves to bits.

19-09-03

I went to university and lost my way, I had written the wrong room number. I have a terrible headache, my feet ache and I had to carry my work from last year. I went to the Mary Ward centre. I am a prat, I prattled, I and another woman are the most experienced writers. Writing is a craft and like any other craft care and attention is needed, so that one does not fall by the wayside.

I need to be still so I can digest, but I am a whirling Dervish. I am going to do a drawing and I can't draw. Every night about this time I write my little diary. I feel so displeased with my writing, I need to write like before, when I was 28 I was writing a novel. I envy people writing.

20-09-03

The voice is gathering himself for the next girl, and the next time I think I will kill him. It's a pity I can't see what he is doing, and in which country. I just feel, that now I did my motherly bit, he'll take wing and fly. He is a slag, he prefers slags, he is a voice which leaves me frustrated and tormented. It is hard when we can't say good bye.

Miss Beyaz was a whore, yet he had elevated her to the heights, plus he groomed her, had sex with her. I need to keep busy, otherwise time does not pass. The voice picks young dancers. He is seriously ruining my health and annoying me.

He needs to settle down but he won't, he elevates women until they fall. I am a fool not to go out all this time. It's late now, 44 years old and still ageing. I read the paper and an article caught my eye about race about colour. About Israel being a question of colour. I agree it is about that, even my life is about race, for I have been discriminated against positively, but when that little girl stole my story because she had polio and I had not, I was discriminated against. My father was too ill to take care of me and, having no one to turn to, I turned to my abuser, and men have abused me ever since.

My sisters made it from the same background; I can't escape 'me'. I can't escape the voices and the despair.

21-09-03

This morning I woke with a sad song on my lips, but the voice objected to the song because a fat woman sang it. He said why did I not sing a song a man sang, and it would prove I was a lesbian etc. Mum had put the TV on and a man was singing soon after the woman, so I sang that.

The voice is rude and obnoxious, I want to go away far away, but I must do my degree and besides, I have no place to go.

I had got away from the first hatred so why can't I get away now? Age, besides I can't do it, last time I lost my memory, this time who knows?

My sisters came and so did Ted and the kids. I washed the dog. I did the shopping with Ziynet and then I mopped up, washed dishes and felt tired. I read Belgin's short story, she can write, and we are proud.

I feel so sleepy I can barely write. Mum and dad argue because Dad won't do anything for himself. Mum keeps on saying your brain will die. Dad ignores her and today he had ten coffees, mum and me made them. I can't stand it and I am going to UEL.

22-09-03

7.10 A.M, I have a cough, a rasping irritating one. I got dressed and fell to working my guts. I'm alone except for the cat that has come into my room. Mother made my bed, treats me like an invalid. I had a three hour lecture, I fell to catching up. Then my bad temper got the better of me and I wanted to kill the voice, except it would be I that would be killed.

But then I have been boring everyone with my ailments, with my uninteresting story for so long that it would just be dandy if I had the guts to do it.

Tomorrow I give work to my class and feel that I am terrified! New people, new things to see, what a dismaying thought after all that time, I am a beginner still.

23-09-03

I hang up the exhibition and waited for the famous teacher to arrive. Except he did not, I asked, and said he was a hero of mine, all maybe untrue. But my work was not commented on. It hung there neglected while I commented on the others, incidentally so did the teacher. I thought her remarks perceptive and she taught me how to look at space more.

Apparently having space gives depth and more meaning to a picture. I am reading a book called Death's Showcase, all about the Jews and art, at the same time as I read, my eye gazed at the waitress reading The Mirror and was reminded of myself when I had been a waitress. Who knows what she might become and she so old.

Then that reminded me of a time when I tried to read the Wasteland, Eliot, and how I could not understand it, and when I asked a customer if he had read and understood it, he said it would take too long to explain. He said that in a dismissive way as if I had been dirt off the streets. He was a well dressed man of stocky build, and then, annoyed, he left. I bet he did not understand the Wasteland either.

Then, years later I heard a reading of it, April is the cruellest month of all, and all that, and I can relate to it. It is about the rattling skeletons, and not as I thought, about the weather, but humanity in particular. But it is all these things. It is so good that it can take years of thought to assimilate to digest it.

Recently I read bits of it in an anthology and it was so beautifully clear that it made me wish I had more time to reread.

24-09-03

Today was a day of reckoning. I pre-emptied my exhibition and everyone went quiet. They did not like it, I could tell. I just wanted to go and paint and destroy the embarrassment of my art. Then I logged on to the internet and cheered up. Susie, my friend went with others and we chatted in the bar. I was too late to have a cup of tea but did have crisps.

We need to do something with music; I chose to do love songs. I emailed chipmunk. I don't know if I got through. My cough has not improved and my tonsils hurt. I am trying to get more money.

26-09-03

Two whole days and I am more settled. My period has come and I feel very dirty. I went to the bar with Anna and Hannah. We had nice hot drinks and before that, Hannah's purse was stolen, and I think she thinks that I did it! We now have lockers and I don't have to carry everything in plastic bags.

I did a painting about aeroplanes, 2 towers and an Arab! I think the new clicks. No one commented on it. Maybe the pathos was lost in the aggressive use of colour?

I tried to work but I felt hampered because I had phone calls to make. The university has taken over my life and my only salvation is to write.

I make crap pictures. I think the group is gelling, but the youth are loud and arrogant, how they remind me of me. How come we don't realize how arrogant we were? Do we all have a memory lapse or do we gloss over our experiences?

I will not get benefit because I am in full time education. I am glad, I was afraid that I would never come off it.

I wrote two poems today, I don't know whether they will be published. I contacted the student paper and got their email address. Also, I gave my email. I acted in a professional manner which pleased me. After all, it still gives me a buzz to be a writer. Growing gracefully old is fun.

Not that I am that old, but it's as if I am a woman whose being a woman is not important. Yet I do all kinds of things like make tea and coffee but not make love! I need it! Not I!

27-09-03

Talking about making tea and being a woman, a woman's work is never done. I am still reading one book after a week. I have glanced through 200 pages and am none the wiser. I have to read more. I loaned some pastels to John, and he sweetly lent me some paint. Gerry was going to phone and he has not.

I am ever so busy. I did dad's insulin, 40 of them. I did that in an hour. Life has become very demanding and productive. I wish I can get my computer, a slow council is working ever so like a tortoise. I'll fail the course and life.

I took Susie to the vet, (not my friend Susie) and Susie is a healthy dog. My stomach is killing me, I have over eaten and the telly was broadcasting best model of the year. There was Kevin Klein looking ragged and gorgeous, he is Turkish. The old man who discovered Kevin changed his name. I wonder if it was something that would have stopped him succeeding.

And there was Miss Beyaz singing without her voice. There were all the beautiful people I can never hope to be. People I'll never be, with no clothes on, looking beautifully groomed. I wish they would go and jump in the lake, but these people the voice calls his wife material, and he'll never learn, the poor thing, has started another affair.

This time I won't say or do anything because I am indifferent to the voice. I just cannot stand the thing.

28-09-03

Today I relaxed, ate. I read Death's Showcase, I just love the title but forget it on a regular basis. I paid for my newspaper, I bought two pens as well. I spelt pens as pence. I am always thinking of money. I can't seem to stretch money. I am going to apply to the Social Security to get Attendance Allowance for mum for looking after dad. Mum is scared about running out of money, and mum off my back will be good.

Mum says she is lazy today. I feel alert but my body has gone to sleep. As if I was spilt into two compartments. My head is separated because suddenly it is free to do, to think, to be.

It is my body that is sick. A lethargy, a disinclination to get going and up. I had two chocolates, that must be the reason, and yesterday I had a cramp on my legs, after sitting I could not get up. I've grown older. My old face stares at me, looking at me with eyes which aren't beautiful or well groomed.

The voice is still looking for female partners for me, and I sometimes want to kill the voice, if I kill the voice will I go to prison?

My life tastes bitter. What with Michael sabotaging the editing of my poetry book a year ago and everything, the momentum of my publishing has gone. But I am free, yet no one is free not really. I found the booklet for the awards and hopefully I can do things, get more money and be more interesting as a consequence. It will take a while to organise myself, I have ideas for the journal which we need to do by Jan.5th. But the trouble is I have no computer. I have nearly read Death's Showcase, I have found it enjoyable.

Night time 11.25

Someone in my head is crucifying me, dissecting every unworthy thought, every look at TV. Even my mother's touching skirt. I am being crucified, yet I can't stop the bastard. He thinks pure thoughts, his mother is dead. He lives all by himself. I feel like murdering him.

Hamlet's father said "Remember me". I am the ghost that did not die, I grow old instead. I don't think I can stand this cat and mouse game. He is all superior, he is smug, and thinks he is virtuous. A sanctimonious pig. There is a demarcation in my heart and it is hurting, I am hurting all over.

He is pigheaded, he has been nodding wisely for the past twenty years. He is like those dolls on windscreens, and he destroys, and he chooses to destroy, because that is what he does best, he does it deliberately. But it is I nodding away, it is me.

Yes I can see that, I have been talking to myself for the past 23 years. I feel like descending into my hole and never getting up. Tomorrow I am going to the UEL and hopefully I'll do some work. I've read Death's Showcase. The art world is opening for me I am going to amount to something.

29-09-03

Went to the UEL and did art theory. I was sat next to John Sheehy. He is very enthusiastic about the book 'Screaming for Air'. He offered me £50 for copies. At first I let it drift, thought he was testing my honesty but realised that he meant it. He wanted those copies. I sent him to the Big Issue. Everybody's enthusiasm is catching.

Then I went to 821 and did my short story reading. I complained that I was not writing things as I had in my twenties. I've lost my way as a story writer. I want to write fiction again. My diary is taking my material. I am churning out stuff most nights.

Then I had to write brief introductions to my paintings, which I did. On Wednesday I have to speak to someone about computers, so I can get one. I phoned on Friday but there had been a fire drill. I spoke about mum getting carers' allowance. It would be one less thing to worry about. Italy has no electricity because a tree was uprooted. Someone in Chechen was poisoned. Turkey wants to elect a new president, all's right with the world.

Mankind is so grasping, me included. If mankind was not so constantly in a grasping mood it would not be surviving.

How do I write more? In England there is no demand for short stories. I can't write the damn things anyway.

30-09-03

I was extremely tired because of bad news, my neighbour died last night. Right next to us, number 48. I could not believe it, God is playing, he was a fat man and died of a heart attack, he was two years older than me. He was a fatherly man whom we gave jobs to. The door we gave him, he didn't do. He complained to the council about a rotten job which someone had done, and saved the house.

He appeared in excellent health. We three will bury the neighbourhood, 2 other people have died nearby, but they were old. They will all be buried next week. The whole neighbourhood is talking about it. We all want to cheer each other up, but there is nothing cheerful about death.

Everyone we know dies, aunts and uncles and cousins. I'm still waiting for my cat to die. I've been waiting several years, I hope not.

1-10-03

Today I was in a creative mood. I could not settle to do anything, I was as if tied onto a tightrope. My teachers were excellent, one sent me to have breakfast, the other gave me excellent advice. Fayzi said something about creativity and the mood I was in was the end product of being creative, and those produce the best works. Just when I was doing it I ran out of paper. I bought 4 A2-paper and still it was not enough, I wished to have more paper. I also ran out of masking tape, I need to get some for tomorrow.

I saw through the window my neighbour's children talking, pale and anxious, all cried out. I wonder when the funeral will be and if we will be invited.

2-10-03

I had woken from anger and mayhem. Maybe it had been the 2 punch drinks which I had had. I sketched a huge head and then coloured it in, and then Gary came and criticised it. The same lines he said, the same marks.

I saw other people's drawings and explained my idea for a video, it has been done before but on aeroplanes, I wanted to do it on the ferry. Gary said it was a brilliant idea. I start filming tomorrow.

Maybe my life is ideal for me to produce stories, but all that I can think of is the wasted years and my regrets. A group of us went to the ICA and saw films about naked people, and people with crossbars trusting each other. Ann and I had a good look, but Sue and Hannah had a drink, Lee went his own way, enjoyed himself, then we went and had a sandwich at Charing Cross. We all had egg which was the cheapest, except for Lee who had ham and tomatoes. Hannah left to look after her cats. I have to begin the journal. I don't know what to write because I write everything in my diary. So I might copy bits from my diary. I need my computer.

Belgin was pleased with me because I was at her book launch. She has had her story published and got paid for it. I am very pleased for her. She can't believe it, and the editor did say that the reason she published it was because it was impersonal.

I am taking the video to college and then I am starting work.

3-10-03

I used the camp recorder, I've started my journal and already I feel better. I have been reading about the women in the surrealist movement. No, it was not only I who had problems with men. Some of these women did nothing but look after family, and if they were young and pretty they were sex objects, but baby sex objects.

I need to rest. I have been busy all day. I have filmed the ferry and the dog, mum, and Hannah. Hannah is a strange girl. She is doing, as her work, plastic taping. She is taping her chair and table, and her dolls and everything she can possibly do. Ann said today she could not afford to buy a camp recorder.

I feel sorry that I bought it, it set me back £500. I have to economise. I can't throw my money away. Next week is Ted's birthday. I suggested we make helva and mum is going to do it. I enjoyed Aydin's story last night, the violence of men, her man, and I had not realised it was so dark. I was shocked with the horror of a horror story.

Dad still has cancer. He has diabetes, blood pressure, schizophrenia and anaemia. He is less difficult but he placed his hand in front of mum's face. They sit side by side, angry and old. I sit opposite because dad smells of urine and I watch them. I rang everyone today.

Jennifer did phone, I think she was pissed off because I had not phoned. I keep on telling her I go to university but she does not understand.

4-10-03

I am in a filthy temper, I have been reading all day and I am highly strung. Jennifer phoned and I am going to see her on Monday at 3 o'clock on the fourth floor café. I am weary of the voice and all my madness, I am weary of life. I think if I want to be forgotten I would end it right here and now.

Uri said I was like one of the surrealists, and now I read them and realise they are all lunatics. I am not a surrealist, although I did copy Frida Kahlo. But then Gary did say "What is the point of copying something already done?"
I want to learn how to paint and draw and hope I can find my voice.

I shouted at mum because she had left an apple to rot. I feel highly strung. I fear what all this leads too. Maybe madness, but who cares if I go mad, I go mad.

5-10-03

Today I was arguing with the voice. No I
don't want to be a man. We argued last night, I
was ill. I spent the day reading about the surrealist
movement. Every word that I read confirmed me
as a woman.

As I argued I caught a chill. I did not lose
my temper. I am a burden on the household.
Yesterday we went out, today we stayed indoors,
shut away from everything. Belgin and mum spoke
on the phone. Then Ziynet phoned, I spoke, she
talked. I respect her; my sister has done things
which demand respect. I had a bath, then read
about Goya, which was in the Guardian. I listened
to Margaret Riley on the radio, her play was
excellent. It taught me what a radio play should
be. I wish I can write like that.

Ziynet's mad sister in law paints as well. I
am mentally impaired. I can do only certain things
at certain time. I have to live with that. The voice
makes me feel tired. No man can be that cruel, no
living thing. I am talking to the self which is vain
and silly. Why?

6-10-03

My demons are now calmer. I've got good
news and bad news. Bad news is I will not be
having two exhibitions, good news is I'll have a
joint exhibition with Sylvia from 28 March to 3

April, also other exhibitions jointly or in groups. So I am all geared up, I have to go and buy canvases.

I saw the Polke exhibition, both when he was a young and playful artist and then when he grew serious. We were at Tate Modern, I don't like the Tate's coffee but the sandwiches are nice.

I met a friend and she told me that John Bird was opening a gallery. I'll phone the Big Issue to see if, or when I've done my exhibition, I can do so again. Dad sleeps a lot. Mum is already complaining that she doesn't get enough money, dad wants more looking after. I finished reading about the surrealist movement. My chest hurts, I don't know if I'm going to make it to my fifties.

7-10-03

Nearly threw myself into the river, but realised in time that the camp recorder would have died too. Two days of work was in it, I don't know if it is good. I think Ann has left. I was so tired today, yet I produced. A different artist is coming to lecture. I'm bringing a fork. Dad is complaining constantly, he is cold.

I read in the paper about an 84 year old who had a bath, then he took the hair dryer to dry himself and set the mattress alight, took the mattress outside and burst a pipe, and set the whole house alight.

Life is full of just such incident. We have not been told when John is being buried. I am an outsider. I will always be an outsider. But last Saturday a woman paid £16 for two loafs. She got her money back but these computers… I'm getting £500 on the 14th. Another scholarship would come in handy.

8-10-03

Mum gets up, washes dad, mops the floor, cleans the bath and I get up to feed all the pets and us, take the dog for a walk. Then race to the bus stop, where I board the bus and read the Guardian. Today I took the camp recorder and lost the cover, luckily not the recorder.

My computer is coming soon, Friday I think, on Friday I have a reading. On Friday all the world is activated like a giant display. I am a part of life. I have a life, I am no longer dead, for a long time I was buried, but no longer so.

I am reading "Camera works", various essays on the camera written in the seventies and eighties. I think of the image I must present to the world, my persona, and I wonder what is it I am studying, when will I create the perfect image? I have endless delights in making the video, but is it any good? Will I be good enough, I read a bit on Sarah Lucas, Moulina and another Iranian woman artist! I have so much to read, it is like my brain is empty and must be filled.

I must write about the voice, the poor thing is being neglected- the same attitude, the same dirt. I am torn between doing good in this world, for example doing work, and just not doing anything to spite the voice. I fear for my sanity. I've so much to do, yet the voice does not help. I nearly said sleep. Every time I speak to a woman the voice does impossible scenarios, casts me in the light of a man. I am a woman, I intend to stay a woman. Every time I speak to a woman or a man it is as if that barrier called normal conversations, normal persons, has been destroyed. I remember last summer and how I nearly stayed in Cyprus. I've forgotten his name and that is as it should be. I must be getting over him because I've forgotten his name.

12-10-03

Mum cooked, I cleaned the house and this kept us busy for most of the morning. The kids came with their parents. We were celebrating Ted's 46 birthday on October 15th. That's big Ted. I took the dog and the children to the park. We all enjoyed ourselves, except for the harassed dog. Even Susie had her moments. Then Susie rushed to Pat's house to complain. I gave Susie treats and so did the children. Susie must have thought it was Christmas.

I have been typing the diary for the past two days and it is exhausting, with all the details of our lives laid bare for everyone to see. But such is life that one has to write about it, it's been written about by many writers, so this one is an effort not to be a great literary work but a work of promise.

I saw the Piano and Odet! Both films are films about their time, about people. I enjoyed them both. Missed Rolf Harris because I was late, I should have been early, but the kids have removed the remote control. Anyway I did not spank them, no getting annoyed, good.

14-10-03

I collected my scholarship cheque. I spoke to Sue, my friend, and then went in search of someone who could print my photos. But I had no luck with that, then came home. I tried to read but slept. Watched Klute, the classic film, but fell asleep through that as well.

I don't know why I am tired, I walk the dog I eat and I sleep all right, it must be my age.
Belgin read tonight, I'll phone her tomorrow or Thursday. We all got lives, even I. So maybe tomorrow I can print the photos, not all, but some?

Today John was buried, I saw the son but I thought I'd leave them. I am not like other people, I kick a fuss for nothing, I did not go to the funeral because I did not know where it was, and did not want to ask for a lift. I asked another neighbour and she said somebody else was giving her a lift.

I saw everyone in their best suits giving John a good bye. I will always be an outsider, I don't know why. I'll be a troubled soul, forever floating with the voice and trying to make some kind of a life. I'd rather die.

18-10-03

It is a quarter to eight in the morning, and my neck aches, I have a heavy cold and I am busy. On Wednesday I saw Romeo and Juliet, which was done at the Young Vic with trapeze artists. The first part was a rollicking do, and in the second part, suddenly, they were serious. I slept.

My films did not work, the camera was incompatible with the gadgets. I am afraid of trying it on my computer in case I upset the delicate machinery. I lost £150.

I need to finish my film on my video camera. I went to the canteen and spoke to everyone, and some star of the show, an upstart woman, began flirting with everyone, including me.

She is on some kind of ego trip. She has all the men on a string.

I am scared but the voice is waiting, I don't want to be a lesbian or to be somebody's ego trip. The voice is encouraging, even going as far as to be encouraging sexual feelings. The trouble is I have no sexual feelings, but a terrible fear, and I can kill the voice. It would be lovely if they did away with the voice, the doctors with their surgical knives?

If I pray hard enough maybe somebody might, for the voice is a frustrating experience with the morals of a con man. The household is waking, I am tired already, but I have an optician's appointment so I can't go back to bed. I have a book which I need to read. I am taking notes. I did a nice screen print yesterday.

19-10-03

Father has started to smoke, he began last night. I feel very calm, as if it's happening but won't hurt me. For the past two days I've been on the phone. I have a reading at the V&A. It is a tremendous honour, I am very pleased. Sarah promised some money. Sarah liked my poems and I'll have ten minutes. I don't know what to read from 'Leaving Turkey'. I'll definitely read The Train. Doctors will be there from the Maudsley (hospital). They did say we'll meet again some day, well, it will be on November 2.

I have been reading and typing my diary. We went to the Chinese place and then Uncle phoned, at first I did not know it was him so I was stand-uppity, but I soon realised my mistake. I called mum, she was on the phone for half an hour.

22-10-03

I had to laugh yesterday when dad said that Mum was being unfaithful with the television. He sat and sat and then came up with it.

Today I went to College and did etching, yesterday I went to college and Graham did my canvas, a huge canvas which used up my 20 foot of wood.

Mum seems fed up. We are going to eat out on Sunday. I and Belgin will pay. My insurance for the camp recorder fell through because I can't do direct debit on my account, so I have to go and pay them directly. Tomorrow I am going on a boat trip. Sarah from the Young Vic is taking us. We 4 students sat and chatted about how young people are arrogant. We older students agreed that they are so. It's nice to know one one is not alone.

26-10-03

It's been three days since I lost my temper with dad and pushed him and he fell onto his seat. I was ever so sorry but at the time I could have killed him, and I would not have felt anything but deep satisfaction. He took my hand and twisted it, but it did not pain me, and it was all because I was due for an injection a week before, so I was a week late for it.

Sometimes I lose it and I don't know what to do about it, but as I have been typing my diary, I can see it building up for a long time. Now I have had my injection I want to sleep all the time. Today we all meet up and are going to the Chinese, but I feel such remorse and guilt, he could have broken my hand and then I would have wasted a whole year. He was more shaken than hurt. His walking got on my nerves. He won't do anything at all, mum has to wash and dress him, and clean after him. He whines all the time and I can't stand it.

But I must not lose it again.

28-10-03

I feel too worn out as if my heart will burst. I now have to help old people. I helped an elderly woman the other day. When I had been ill some years back and was scared of children, I had to help children. I went to the doctor the other day and told the doctor that I pushed dad.

The doctor looked into my soul and was shocked to the core, absolutely shocked as if he had seen me do murder or mayhem, and I was embarrassed and shocked too, but what to do with my temper? I now have to have injections every two weeks instead every three.

Angie, poor thing, thought I was doing well and was happy, but the doctor gave him one shattering look for being so much in the past. I wish I could turn back the clock. Angie said I could have broken dad's ribs. Mum took my side of the story, she actually said that I did not mean it. The trouble was that I did mean it at the time, but am now awash with guilt. Poor mum.

Anyway, since yesterday I have slept, and the voice is a voice, and a kiss is just a kiss, and a smile is just a smile, and whatever next I don't know.

29-10-03

I went and acted in a play, not my own, the nurse in Romeo and Juliet. Hope I did justice to the role, had to be protective towards Juliet. There were twelve of us and we all acted with enthusiasm. Went to college and started my sculpture. Also saw my counsellor for the first time. She is coming on Sunday for my big day.

I came home and slept, after I emptied the bin and walked the dog I felt very tired. I am going back to bed now. It is nearly twelve and the voice is less active thank God. Although he still has a word it is I who am strong. This illness is nothing like anything even though my arthritis is playing up, so is my blood pressure, schizophrenia is terrible.

Schizophrenia destroys the whole fabric of life, and makes me a slave to the doctor and the nurse, and then the doctor the nurse, and so it goes on.

30-10-03

Had a really rewarding but draining day, a day filled with so many ups. The book 'Screaming for Air' was printed, and so at last it was what the vendors had dreamed of, what they had wanted. The vendors took it all so to heart as if their whole lives had been turned into gold. That was my reward.

I had invited people from the university, but they did not come, but the vendors invited people from Groundswell who gave us the money, and was so influential in being so good to us. Groundswell came, and so had John Petherbridge, whose example had made the choosing of the poems so easy.

I thank them all. Francis was there and so was Fiona, and so was John and Gerry, and Fabini and Jason, and I read, and so did they, and it was a wonderful night.

At the university I have started a figure which I am going to put paper on, sugar paper. I felt tired and drained all day, yet it was a wonderful day. A worthwhile one, when I went to the wood work class Paul did say "Was I not doing too much"? One more reading and I am done for the week.

31-10-03

I have nothing to lose, I am a human being with nothing to lose, this gives a sense of freedom, a sense of falling from air as if one is a ball. Feelings akin to torture is gripping me I have been mutilated, my brain has been burnt and my concentration is slipping as if I am a sieve. I have been bounced round as if I am a kitten who is cute. I've lost my senses and I have recovered and lost it again, and I don't intend to lose it again.

I feel a terrible weakness in my heart, as if my heart would burst. I was watching Yul Brynner, he was with a blonde and they fall for each other. I remembered my night twenty years ago and how it had been my night. It had been a turning point which had made me a loser. I never want to remember it, because the person that I became is from that night, but it was a painful birth. I kissed someone and the silly voice took exception. That was when the voice became dominant in my life; it would not let me be.

I can't fight the voice, I want to but can't. The poor me that became a loser was from that night. Not long afterwards my short story appeared in a magazine, but I never wrote so freely again. The voice took over, it became dominant. I allowed it to torture me all those years because I grew ill.

Now it's too late to change, too late. The ever same years, and me and the voice hating one another, loathing one another, but living together in the same head, same skull, but never separating because we can't, and mankind has it good because they can separate.

The hateful voice won't go away and won't be a man, it is not a man. The voice's heart I will tear apart, like he has torn my heart.

4-11-03

I saw a counsellor and spoke about what the voice is doing, we ended up talking about father, and how he had tried to kill mum all those years ago. John and I spoke for a long time and I enjoyed it. Hannah was out of sorts, she is a student in my class, and my friend. She said she had spent four hours travelling on the bus and in the end she lost her temper. Mad you see, what can one do with traffic? One has to read or one goes mad. Hannah also said she will skip the lectures on Mondays, as she finds it tiring.

I had a similar thing to say to the Young Vic too. I had found the Young Vic too stressful, my dear. I spoke to a 23 year old Turkish Cypriot girl. We said absolutely foul things about our situations, which she finds comfortable, her mother dusting and cleaning, and her mother's divorce. It was one of those talkative spells I have. On Sunday the event never happened. I went, yes, but I could not find them. So my counsellor came and I had soup, and my anger just became lodged in my stomach.

Last night I read a bit of my short story at the Poetry Café, and had an exhibition in the Crypt. It all made up for the Sunday's disappointment. The Postal strike was to blame, because I did not know where to go.

6-11-03

I finished my short story and began to write my essay, and then I waited for the technician, and waited and waited, but then he said tomorrow. I want to stretch my canvases. Spoke to everyone and went to the second and third year exhibitions. I think we are better artists although they are technically more brilliant. One of their paintings was superb.

I just realised what the voice is, he is a fascist. The Nazis exterminated the Jews and he buries me alive. I can just see him with high heels and a whip. A homo to the core, and he makes me sick.

I nearly fell down the boats' stairs I was trying to climb up, and was trying to avoid a woman because the voice said I fancied her, and I did not. So we argued when the boat docked and I nearly fell. I was forced to stand there behind the woman feeling foolish, and waited to get off.

Then I caught a bus to Woolwich, avoiding people playing on the bus stop, which was not in use the previous night, and I was not going to see if it was in use tonight. I was fearful they would take my money because they were playing, and this man was watching them, two men and a woman. Were they a gang or just my frenzy? I did not stay to find out. One can't be too careful these days.

I went to the bus and started to read my paper. More about Mr Brown and the Prime Minister quarrelling, and an interesting article about fatherhood should mellow Brown. Blair's heart scare was a Godsend to him. Then Prince Charles and his dodgy sexuality, I just love reading the paper. Poor Iraq and its people, why did war start? Now I am going to bed.

9-11-03

Sisters, Ted, and the children are coming today. I have slept but yesterday I went to the theatre and saw His Girl Friday, and was there just in time for the start of the show at the National, one is allowed to be a bit late.

Today my heart is a bit sick. I write about my feelings and my heart a lot, but the voice is holding my heart like a vice, and I just can't seem to escape the consequence of the voice.

12-11-03

Today was less bizarre than creepy yesterday. Yesterday I could have sworn I saw giant white-dressed figures, and heard a screech saying Suzy. Even now I am mad, stark staring mad. So today we put up the show, we painted the walls of the university, and conversed in canteens, and life is interesting. Hard work is interesting, I am terrified by my blisters, I can't walk.

The group that met in the canteen had one thing in common, we all want to finish our degree, and are passionate about it.

Men seek me out, and I talk, God how I talk, and there is always the fear that the voice will drive a wedge in it. I am always looking over my shoulder to see what is coming behind me.

Everyone is going to bed, I am dressed in my night dress, and I am writing this. Yesterday is in the past. I am no longer mad. The voice is under control. I am in control of myself. Mary has taken my book and won't give it to me. Mary is my Counsellor.

14-11-03

Days like these when all I do is sleep. It is necessary, but I wish I was strong so that I can stay awake, the voice keeps on saying he is gay, he slept with the highest and the lowest. I want to scream but there is only nothing.

Today passed like this and yesterday. I had a tutorial and Fazil told me my screen print needed more work. Fazil is a good teacher, then we all went to an exhibition of the third year, and they are really different to the first year. They select more, more organic.

What will my exhibition with Sylvia be like? I handed my essay to be criticised, and today I just crashed out.

15-11-03

I went to the dentist today and paid fifteen pounds, but mum paid most of it. Mum and I had agreed that she would pay. The dentist made a long face, "trauma and the like, gums bad, hospital might be a good idea." They gave mum an appointment after six months. I wonder if it gets better as one gets older?

There is a thief masquerading as a policeman. I live in fear, I have a good deal of worldly goods and I don't want to lose them.

Dad was waiting for us at the bus stop, and we all went to our Chinese place where we eat and don't pay a lot. I could not have a coke, so had tea and orange juice. I hate the voice, it is like he does not want me, nor I him. He hates me, what we had was a string-along someone.

When I was trying to do the reading he knew where to go, and did not go, on purpose, just because I wanted money. He is always a scum and I hate scum.

I have to gurgle five times in salt water; I wonder when I'll be dead? Salt and blood pressure don't mix. The dentist knew I have blood pressure so maybe it is safe.

17-11-03

After three days in bed I am now recovered. Today I did a bit of this and a bit of that. My mouth aches so I made a dental appointment for tomorrow.

I've argued my points with the voice. I've decided the voice makes me tired as if it is doing it on purpose to make me ill.

My tutor made suggestions for the essay, and I've got to get the catalogue and see about the Viola exhibition. I've decided I'll go on Saturday. On Saturday Roger is coming but he can do it himself. The essay is far more important. I have to get titles of the paintings etc.

The voice is a real bastard, apparently not gay, but doesn't seem to be interested in dull and unattractive woman. The chap next door is too young and the one in college is too old, and his breath smells. I sound exactly like the voice.

20-11-03

Today is father's 69th birthday. I went to university and had to change where I paint, it is lovely up there. I feel very happy. It is on the second floor. Today I took down the exhibition. I realize that two of my paintings will decay, I did not prime them.

I took everything upstairs. I was helped by a kind gay chap whom I told I had a heart condition. I milked the situation, but I got a table and a chair. I told the voice off.

24-11-03

Today I went and saw the Turner Prize exhibition, liked it. I said Grayson should win, he is the one that did pottery and paintings, and a cross dresser too. The whole of the 1st year were there. Then we had a discussion and later we saw actual Turner exhibition. I just love the sunsets and the way he captures light and shade.

Then I met a friend and we had coffee. Later I went to Jaime's exhibition, it was terribly good. Collins said he thought my paintings were beautiful. The exhibition will run to three months and the pictures sold, the new owners can take immediately, and are to be replaced, and so it goes on.

For 5 days there was no hot water. I smelt of urine and sweat, I tried to have a bath but boiling the water does not add up to enough, not on the gas stove. Well today it was fixed. Mother had a bath.

Belgin came to the exhibition, and helped with serving and washing up. I introduced her to people. She mixes well. She is confident. I broke two glasses.

25-11-03

I got up and rushed like mad, was late for university because I had to phone the chiropodist who starts at 9.30am. I also collected mum's pension. I got to the university with all the rest of the people. I have not done any work today on the essay, but have done lots of painting and my journal. I was on the radio today. This gave me a lovely feeling, although I could not hear it properly and had to switch off.

All my friends left the room except for Mary who is my counsellor. Anyway the counselling session went off well and the voice was not active. Then the voice began.

It is a mischievous voice. It will destroy me. I'll die, but it seems to be me.

27-11-03

The voice was very much in the wrong today. A teacher came to my rescue. She said things to reassure me. She said she looked at boots, and pants and socks, and stockings, their textures. She raved over a boot a girl was wearing. I am an artist so I must look at things. I look at clothes, I look at bottoms, I make comparisons with women about bottoms. I am always on the look out for an idea for a painting.

The voice should have been an actor. He would have petrified the audience. He is still in love with Miss Beyaz. He, poor thing, wants to have children, not by me, but some woman. He took the only man I cared for and left me in the company of sheep. I don't love J, God help me, I tried. I have ceased loving Oktay. I am now heart free, fancy free.

I'll never love again. I'll explain, when I was 24 I loved a man more than life itself and then the voice got rid of him. He disappeared. I waited and waited, I had a huge breakdown in consequence. My lover never came back and I am left with these spineless men. Now there is no one about only me, and the shadows forcing me into destruction.

29-11-03

I wonder if what I've written will be of any relevance to anyone? Will I be read? As anyone can see, I've passed through fire. The voice is broken, his lover was on television and I could see her wit has deserted her.

I don't need to be vindictive but I am I am also a crazy bitch. Today not much has happened, I've read the paper and a book, I am going to see Mathew Collings on television. Read his 'What Is Art', enjoyed it. Some of his opinions are perceptive. His discovery of the light switch installation in 1999, before the Turner exhibition, very perceptive.

I've nearly completed 'Nothing Sacred' and I feel a crude sense of achievement. I hope nothing bad happens to anyone of us.

Minutes tick, and a sleepy feeling comes over me like I am doing too much, and it is as if I am dying. The voice is chiding me, but yes, I am moving towards death. The only thing that's binding to this life is mother, father, and the dog. My cat is almost dead. So as the minutes tick I am moving towards the vacuum. I feel very sleepy. I must get to bed and sleep.

1-12-03

Today I was aroused really aroused by a man called D. I think he felt the same way. I hope the voice don't stop it because it is good. The voice was, as usual, thinking about himself, and his lack of biological link. He wants a baby.

I saw D and he was nothing to look at, but we chatted and then after chatting for some time we realised that we were turned on. We said common things, chit chats, yet there was a difference in the way we said these things, it was as if every pore of me had been alerted.

Today our lecturer was ill. We all fell to a holiday mood. I spoke to S and fear that due to family problems the poor kid won't pass. We have to submit an essay and a journal, he has not even begun.

2-12-03

Today I've gone right to the bottom. Mary, my counsellor saw me, and I hope it won't recur. I think it's my period, anyway, after an hour I was strong enough to paint. Will I ever be free?

I painted a huge canvas; it was my father in a hat done four times. No, D.

4-12-03

My period, I think, is coming. I am sane, thank God. Already tomorrow is my injection. I saw D. today. He walked in hurt silence, I am not involved. Later I talked to my tutor and did a lot of work. I also went to Jaime's but could not paint on top of oils. I have to paint six pictures by January.

I feel very alive, as if all my limbs are there, it's painful and little things make me happy. But I've ceased noticing things. Why? I don't know, it is as if I am a bitch, but do not want to be.

6-12-03

I have talked to mum, about the grant money, how we are going to pay it back. Mum is worried in case things happen. I had to reassure her.

I walk the dog every day and usually it is a pleasure, but today Susie started growling. The other dog owner was amused, because Susie is small and the other dog was huge. I was angry with Susie. The park was muddy, and drizzle was pouring, and I was enjoying the cold. The mud had soaked right through my shoes and a neighbour's words echoed in my brain, "Wellington boots, that is what you need!"

I spoke harshly to a friend yesterday because she was talking too much and would not let me get on with it. We were in and out of the canteen and no work done. I was angry with her and said so, "I have no children, my work is all I have!"

7-12-03

Today and yesterday I just primed the canvases and rested, but yesterday I worked till eight, and today I woke up at 9.a.m. I was rested. The kids came over with sisters. Belgin treated us to a 3 course meal, it was lovely.

Then we came home and I went upstairs with Roger, and we got on the internet. Roger typed my name and up it came, with details of a reading which I had not gone to, and my very first book.

Then more again with the voice. I might even be a battered wife. My ego is nothing to the voice, and I am so tired. The voice does not want me to write about it, very wise of him. I read the paper a bit. Then saw the Turner prize. I am glad that Grayson won. I wish I could win too!

9-12-03

When love dies it is so hard to be in the same situation, the same room, and the same person. I think that is why people change persons so frequently. Love is like a will a wisp. The fragility of love is underestimated.

I am the same person but a part of me hates me, and I hate that person. The dog gets scared if I talk to the voice on the Common. I notice that it gets naughty when I talk to the voice.

I had such a headache this evening. I feel like an adult now. I went to an exhibition, the talked to the radio people. I've been on the radio twice and might be on for a third time. I might wheedle my way over in the New Year. I wrote a little poem.

I painted a picture by using ink and water and water colours. Tomorrow I'll see my Counsellor.

10-12-03

Today I experienced such bitterness, mother's milk had gone sore and turned into gore.

I had those words in my mind, life and its bitter sweetness. Today I am going to a party, where anything might happen. Nothing did, I was my boring self.

I had to see if anything had changed, I have not changed. I have remained the same, literally the same. The same feelings of trying to escape the voice, only to be trapped like a butterfly.

12-12-03

Yesterday all my friends got together and dissected the Christmas party. One of my friends had brought flashing knickers. She won a prize with that, the prize was a day out in a gallery. One of the girl's had got so drunk, she had to be carried to her room. The tutor asked how she was, one of my friends reassured him. So a merry Christmas had been had by all except me, the sobersides.

I too want to let my hair down, but the dreary voice in my head won't let me. I too want to be loved before it is too late, why should not I? I am a human being. I get so lonely sometimes, I want so much to touch a man, a man who don't play games.

13-12-03

Today I had a reading and a college reunion. I got up at 7 A.M, because it was raining I could not take my dog to the Common, it had to be on the road. Then had breakfast, and without reading the paper or anything raced to Custom House station. I found it easier than the V&A, More approachable, at least I had all the forms and documents on me, it was the third floor and Ken Livingstone was there.

I had a belated cup of tea and, as it was on the house, another and another. Then I had to go to the toilet. I must have drunk a whole bottle of mineral water, so I was popping up and down for about an hour. I went for the last time 5 minutes before the gig.

I read my poem and it was over. I played the shakers as well. I also spoke to Ken Livingstone about the 'top up' fees. How it is wrong to be in debt for the rest of one's life.

I also listened to a brilliant lecture by a man in a wheelchair who spoke about the negatives of being disabled. There is a whole scenario in films and things which implies to be disabled is to be self willed. If only it were true. No I don't will myself to be disabled, I would give anything not to hear the voice, and my mum, is she willing herself to be disabled, and dad too? It is like an elderly person who wills themselves to be old.

No, this diary will have no happy ending, no conclusion. It will be going on, and I guess people will form their own conclusions about me. I am ending the diary before the festive season, because getting fat, and eating like a pig, is what we all do.

I'll end the diary now.

END OF VOLUME ONE

Printed in the United Kingdom
by Lightning Source UK Ltd.
128289UK00001B/39/A